AF240869

THE SADNESS BUSINESS

Patrick Landman

THE SADNESS BUSINESS

Max Milo
ESSAIS-DOCUMENTS

Max Milo Editions

Collection Essais - documents, Paris, 2023

www.maxmilo.com

ISBN : 978-2-31501-148-3

In memory of Jean Clavreul and Roger Misès
To Eva, Quentin, Chloe and to those to come...

Introduction

How can the *Diagnostic and Statistical Manual of Mental Disorders*, or DSM, have the power to manufacture lunatics and one day label you as mentally ill when you are well ensconced in a legitimate sense of normalcy?

First published in 1952 in the United States under the aegis of the American Psychiatric Association (APA), the first version of the DSM listed 60 mental disorders. Today, there are more than 350 disorders listed in the DSM-5. If DSM-1 and DSM-2 were still in line with the clinical psychiatric approach, the following versions have gone against it. Hence the increase in the number of disorders listed and the need today to demonstrate the limits and dangers of the DSM.

In some American states, nearly 25% of school-age children are treated for attention deficit disorder with or without hyperactivity; in France, this figure is currently less than 3% but it is constantly increasing; one French person in five takes psychotropic drugs. The responsibility for these facts of psychiatry, which I would call "DSM psychiatry", is very important, and I could multiply the examples. But figures are not enough in themselves, they must be interpreted correctly. It can be argued, for example, that these figures reflect a better scientific knowledge of mental illnesses, better prevention with earlier detection, in a word an improvement in the field of mental health. I will show that this is not the case.

As a child psychiatrist and a psychiatrist, I have long been reluctant to consider that the DSM could have an impact of this magnitude. I did not use it in my practice for years and it is only recently that I started to take an interest in it. Others in France had been more perceptive, perceiving the importance of the DSM, the change in mentalities that it embodies, the anthropological consequences that it accompanies and the new paradigms that it uses. For my part, I lived with the idea of the "French exception" which, in my opinion, conferred a sort of protection of both professional ethics and good practice applied to patients. This French exception was based on three pillars. The first pillar is the psychodynamic tradition, which comes from psychoanalysis, from Lacan in particular, and which gives a preponderant place to listening, to the history of the subject, to speech, while seeking psychopathological explanations without prejudging the cause of mental illness. The second pillar is the French - and even European - psychiatric clinical tradition, which is schematically based on differentiated structures called *neuroses, acute and chronic psychoses, perversions,* and *dementias.* These categories are fundamental for clinical identification, for the practitioner's understanding and for the action to be taken. In this context, for example, the term "madness" - apart from the use of a substance or a state of dementia - is reserved for the single category of psychosis. The last pillar is due to the initiative of Professor Roger Misès who, because of his dual training as a psychoanalyst and child psychiatrist, understood in the 1980s the danger of the DSM, especially for child psychiatry[1]. He then set up a working group that set about building a French Classification of Mental Disorders in Children and Adolescents (CFTMEA). The vast majority of French child psychiatrists used this classification, which they recognized[2].

I had bought the French version of the DSM-3. This book, a worldwide bestseller, fell out of my hands. I came out of this reading reinforced in the idea that such an

---

1. Roger Misès (1924-2012) also developed a "new psychiatric clinic", based on multidisciplinary work involving educators, psychologists, pedagogues, psychiatrists, nurses, etc. His main concept is the institutional cure.

2. There are two main types of classification which correspond to two types of approach. On the one hand, the classifications that we will call "clinical classifications" for simplicity's sake, which are based on traditional clinical reasoning, such as the CFTMEA, and on the other hand, the atheoretical classifications such as the DSM or the classification of the World Health Organization (WHO) - the International Classification of Diseases (ICD) - which, in its tenth version, is similar to the DSM.

Introduction

indigestible and superficial work, in spite of its claim to be built like an expert system, could never supplant the clinical tradition. I was wrong.

Several events gradually changed my perception of the impact of the DSM.

First of all, my contact with the faculty of medicine made me realize that students and interns were being trained in the DSM and not in the classical clinic: in other words, that the DSM was becoming the main, and sometimes the only, reference for the teaching of this medical discipline that is psychiatry. Just as in politics there had been the "Mitterrand generation", in psychiatry the "DSM generation" was emerging, for which psychoanalysis was a method like any other, or even an archaism, but in any case not a central reference.

Then, a decisive event: my renewed contact with the psychiatric institution via the Jean Macé Establishment, in Montreuil sous Bois, after several years of exclusive liberal practice. This contact allowed me to measure the growing influence of medical economics on the life of these institutions, which did not improve the quality of patient care. I also had the opportunity to measure during meetings, and in their minutes, to what extent the language used in the DSM was taken up by many practitioners, and especially by the health and medico-social administration.

And then there were the screening campaigns for "future delinquents" starting in kindergarten, which rightly scandalized many child professionals and citizens; they are also linked to the DSM because it is not content to make random diagnoses - such as Oppositional Defiant

Disorder[3], or Attention Deficit Hyperactivity Disorder -, but proves to be fixist, with no evolutionary conception of the diagnosis, which is no longer a simple snapshot at a given moment, but rather a final label. It therefore biases the epidemiological studies on which these screening campaigns are based.

Finally, I found, with statistics to back it up, that the DSM was the basis for the increasingly widespread prescription of amphetamines to children, first in the United States and the United Kingdom, but also in France to a lesser extent.

All this data led me to take action with a few others against the single thought of the DSM.

The growing medicalization of affects, especially sadness, which is part of our daily psychic life but whose excessive pathologization is symptomatic of the drift and malaise of our culture - this is what I wanted to express in choosing the title of my book -, the increasingly widespread practice of overdiagnosis and finally the increasingly frequent recourse to psychotropic drugs: these three elements catalyze, in a way, the factory of the insane. It is obvious that its causes are multiple and complex, but the DSM plays a significant role in what can be called a major trend.

In the days when Henri Ey and Jacques Lacan were interns, it was written in the ward of the Hôpital Sainte-

---

3. Oppositional Defiant Disorder is defined by the DSM as a pattern of hostile or defiant behavior toward authority figures that goes beyond typical childhood behavior.

Anne: "Not everyone becomes crazy. This sentence, which is highlighted, demonstrates the relevance of clinical reasoning based on the search for psychic structures: a neurotic does not become psychotic, even if he has to face contrary or tragic circumstances, and a psychotic who is stabilized does not become neurotic. If one accepts that the psychic structures are valid, then the reader can rightly feel reassured that he has a sufficient degree of normality, or in psychiatric language, that he is a normal neurotic without troublesome symptoms. He has nothing to fear, he will not go mad.

Unfortunately, everything is not as simple as it seems. First of all, the psychic structures only correspond to clinical categories, they are not validated by any biological marker of any kind, they are not scientifically validated. Moreover, they are not defined in a sufficiently precise way to reach a consensus and a fortiori unanimity. They present borderline forms which, for some, are transitional or intermediate forms and for others, additional categories. The category of *borderline* states was thus invented. This vagueness was one of the arguments put forward by the promoters of the DSM to justify their refusal to take structures into account and to opt for atheorism in their methodology, which they hoped would be more reliable because it avoided partisan quarrels as well as doctrinal options that were sometimes speculative and often irreconcilable.

But if the "classic" clinic does not offer a high-level guarantee to differentiate madness from non-madness and the atheorism of the DSM manufactures madmen, how can one believe a psychiatric diagnosis or know if one is really suffering from a mental illness? All the modifications in relation to the norm that are observed in mental illnesses, and which are real, must be considered as correlations and not as causes. That is to say, for example: if, in such and such a mental illness, one observes a modification of one or more biological constants or a cerebral modification, the interpretation at the present time cannot affirm that this is the cause of the illness, but rather that this or these modifications are correlated to the illness. To try to be even clearer, I would take the example of fever, which is correlated with very different syndromes or illnesses without being the cause, but with a characteristic that does not exist in psychiatry: fever is a sign that testifies to a reaction of the organism and therefore certainly to a pathological process; however, the anomalies of the organism and its physiology observed in psychiatry have failed until now to play the role of a sign

After these remarks on the lack of scientificity of the classifications of mental illnesses, we must judge these classifications according to criteria other than science. The DSM is responsible for a considerable increase in the number of false positives, in particular "false lunatics", thereby contradicting the basic rules of the medical art. The usual clinical criteria are not above reproach, far from it, but they are much more demanding than the DSM method, which is expeditious and opens the way to prescribing medication often too quickly and inappropriately.

We can help in a less invasive way than medication, avoiding the risk of making patients dependent and causing sometimes irreversible side effects. Using the DSM to make a diagnosis is very convenient, within everyone's reach - which is a considerable advantage in these times of shortage of psychiatrists; but the answer it provides is most often medication. However, the vast majority of patients who consult a psychiatrist, and a fortiori a general practitioner, do not present a severe mental pathology, but rather existential difficulties or crises, problems of adaptation in the broadest sense, moments of professional or sentimental rupture, particularly painful bereavements, educational or couple difficulties, etc. Faced with these demands, it is very satisfying to be able to offer a response that relieves, calms or anaesthetizes anguish or moral pain: this is the purpose of prescribing psychotropic drugs, whose short-term success is undeniable, but questionable in the long term. On the other hand, an instrument such as the DSM makes it possible to provide a rational framework, to constitute these existential complaints as mental disorders and to avoid practitioners the prolonged confrontation with the care of patients. This is one of the reasons why the consumption of psychotropic drugs is at such a high level in France.

The DSM is not the only one involved, of course, but it has a responsibility of its own. It is increasingly used as a reference by the social security system - for example, it has sent general practitioners a *guideline* on major depressive disorder which is modelled on the DSM and encourages them to screen for depressive states in a few minutes using a structured interview. Moreover, the

DSM lends itself very well by its form and its method to a policy of standardization which requires an accelerated evaluation of clinical situations and a homogenization of practices.

The DSM was originally designed for research; its application to practice came from a contagion between the field of clinical drug trials and daily practice. A patient in everyday psychiatric practice is far from being the same as an individual included in research on the efficacy of a drug. It is not obvious to me that psychiatric patients should all be treated in the same way without taking into account their singularity.

For all these reasons, I consider the DSM to be detrimental to health.

1. The new factory of fools

In the popular representation, the madman is the one who sees things that do not exist for the others, who hears voices that the others do not hear, who says things that the others judge incoherent, shocking for the common sense or without relationship with what they perceive of the reality. There exists in everyone and very early on a naïve opinion of what psychic normality is, which is neither entirely spontaneous nor entirely constructed by culture. This opinion resists, in my opinion, all the theories, it is anchored in each one of us and it testifies to a certain common sense. It could be expressed in these terms: psychic normality exists. But as soon as it is a question of giving a precise definition or contents to this psychic normality which is apprehended naively, one runs up against very great, even insurmountable difficulties. Nevertheless the "normal" man confronted with a "crazy" neighbor will feel an affect of fear, rejection or compassion testifying of a feeling of rupture.

Madness has always been frightening, not only because of its association with the irrational, but also because it is the place where anxieties are projected. But it interests everyone, it concerns everyone. Since Philippe Pinel, the great French alienist who, according to the legend, freed the insane from their chains[4], the madness is medicalized, it is considered as a disease, the insane are not any more assimilated to the criminals and locked up in the same places. This transformation did not however make the fear of madness disappear, which was transformed into a fear of mental illness. Moreover, there is still a confusion between madness and criminality, even if it is not validated by facts and statistics. It persists because its roots do not lie in simple reason: rationality does not fight on equal terms with preconceived ideas and prejudices, especially if the political discourse favors these worries and confusions.

The fear of madness associated with its over-dimensioned danger in the collective imagination is at the origin of phenomena of separation, exclusion, and even segregation with regard to the "mad". This separation between the insane and the others takes on more or less visible aspects socially but has never disappeared,

---

4. Philippe Pinel (1745-1826) was in favor of abolishing the irons that shackled the mentally ill. He was one of the first to consider that the "insane" could be cured by dialogue and to abolish drug treatments and bloodletting.

because no society can accept to tolerate a complete indifferentiation between the insane and the others; all societies have principles of regulation and elimination of non-standard behavior. Faced with this observation, there are those who accommodate this barrier of separation for multiple reasons, among which the feeling that their normality is reinforced, and there are those who do not accept it. It is within this second heterogeneous group that different approaches have been proposed to reduce this gap between the insane and the others.

Normality and madness

First, there was the political approach to madness. It reached its peak in the 1960s and 1970s: madness would be the result of social injustice, the insane would be a category of oppressed people, they would collectively have their place among the victims of the capitalist system. Mental alienation would not be very different from social alienation, it would be a particular expression of it. This theory of mental illness as a non-reality gave rise to anti-psychiatry and the opening of asylums, leading in many cases to perverse results: the sick are returned to their families, who bear the burden, or end up on the street.

The failure of anti-psychiatry can be interpreted in two ways. Either the liberation of the insane was premature because it can only happen at the moment of the liberation of the whole society, of the rupture with the capitalist system; or the political conception of insanity

1. The new factory of fools

is inadequate because there would be a reality of insanity that cannot be eliminated by political measures. The positive posterity of anti-psychiatry is found in what is called post-psychiatry.

The psychoanalytical approach to madness also tends to reduce the gap between the insane and the normal. Freud explained that everyone in the course of their development goes through a phase of perversion, the famous "polymorphic infantile perversion[5]". For her part, Melanie Klein affirmed that normal psychic development went through phases that resembled point by point the modalities of functioning of severe psychoses. In other words, we are all former perverts and former psychotics. For psychoanalysis, normality seems to be assimilated to the power to overcome these archaic stages that threaten us during any regression. There would be the idea for psychoanalysis, if not of a hierarchy between madness and normality, at least of a progress. These perverse and psychotic modalities are never entirely erased, they persist in the normal psyche - in the unconscious - and can quite reappear during significant events. It is the fear of the reappearance of our own infantile madness which would be at the origin of our fear of the mad: the mad resemble us, or rather resemble too much our unconscious and threaten our feeling of normality, which is part of our identity. Psychoanalysis has modified the concep-

---

5. It is a question for the child of discovering himself, as well as discovering the world through his sexual impulses, not genital: the sucking, the satisfaction of the various erogenous zones, etc.

tion of psychic normality but has not called into question the very idea of normality.

These two approaches, anti-psychiatry and psychoanalysis, have in common, to varying degrees, to establish a link between madness and normality in a movement that starts from normality to conclude in the extreme that "the mad are normal". Since the 1980s, we have witnessed an opposite evolution with the DSM, which can be summarized as follows: normals are crazy. The result and the starting hypotheses are not the same as in the previous approaches and, above all, if anti-psychiatry and psychoanalysis only affected a minority, the DSM will have consequences on practically the whole population.

The DSM as recognition of the identity of the psychiatrist

Among the proponents of a marked separation between the insane and the others, psychiatrists were overrepresented. This separation validated their profession. They were considered, or considered themselves, to be specialists in madness; which implies that madness exists, that it is distinct from the norm like any pathological state, that it can be named and possibly broken down into different subsets, and above all treated. If madness becomes indistinct from the norm, the psychiatrist disappears, unless he becomes an anti-psychiatrist or a psychoanalyst. It is therefore easy to understand why psychiatrists have held on to the dividing line between madness and normality. On the other hand, psychiatrists

1. The new factory of fools

are also subject to a kind of segregation. If the insane are set apart, so are psychiatrists, their specialty not being scientific, or not as scientific as the rest of medicine, and dealing with vague questions, with a social tone.

These professional parameters were to have a great influence at the turn of the 1970s, when the team charged by the American Psychiatric Association (APA) with revising the classification of mental illnesses, our famous DSM, was set up to develop version 3. From the outset, several trends emerged within the *task force*. An anti-segregationist tendency, for example, with the justified refusal to consider homosexuality as a mental pathology; a scientific tendency that believed or banked on the imminent discovery of biological markers attesting to the organic etiology of the main mental illnesses; and an empiricist tendency that consisted of rejecting psycho-pathological and psychoanalytical concepts as abstract, speculative and idealistic, and of seeking a founda-tion validated by evidence. All of these orientations converged, unbeknownst to the protagonists, to arrive at a classification that would tend to include the vast majo-rity of the population in the clutches of mental illness, to the satisfaction of the pharmaceutical industries.

The art of categorizing our behaviors

In order to make a classification more reliable, it was necessary to remove everything that complicates agree-ment between practitioners, and therefore everything that may appear subjective. The best method for determining pathologies is therefore to stick as much as possible to a summary description of immediately observable behaviours and then to group them into "disorders". If mental illnesses can be reduced to an association of behaviours, unrelated to personal history or environment, the criterion of normality will depend on the cut-off point at which a behaviour or association of behaviours is considered to be pathological in its intensity, frequency or duration. However, it has been found that, from one revision to the next, the DSM has shown a downward trend in inclusion thresholds, a greater "flexibility" in the criteria separating normal from pathological.

Version 5, released in the spring of 2013, is no exception to this trend. It is true that it does not seem to include more disorders a priori than its predecessor, but some of them are likely to include a considerable number of subjects, especially children. The former chairman of the DSM-4 *task force*, Professor Allen Frances[6], has focused his rejection of DSM-5 on the idea that it is becoming urgent and absolutely necessary in the field of mental health to "save normality". In fact, normality is virtually non-existent in the DSM. For example, if someone continues to be very distressed on the sixteenth day of a bereavement, he or she is liable to be prescribed psychotropic drugs in the name of a supposed evolutionary risk of the bereavement towards severe depression. This evolution is logical, because if we look only at the

---

6. FRANCES (Allen), *Saving Normal: An Insider's Revolt Against Out-of-Control Psychiatric Diagnosis, DSM-5, Big Pharma, and the Medicalization of Ordinary Life*, New York, William Morrow/HarperCollins Publishers, 2013.

behavioral dimension, there is little difference between a state of mourning and a major depressive state. We also know that normal mourning can evolve into pathological mourning; but for this to happen, several conditions were classically required, in particular duration; to make this duration disappear or to reduce it to so little seems to me to be symptomatic of everything that can be denounced about the DSM-5: medicalization of affects, over-diagnosis, over-prescription, confusion between the precautionary principle and true prevention.

The drug stranglehold

So be it, but two arguments can be raised. First: You warn us about the fear of being wrongly included among the insane, of suffering the side effects of inappropriate prescriptions, of becoming dependent on the action of chemicals or of being forced to increase the doses to obtain the same effects; but after all, it is an individual choice, we are not obliged to consume these drugs, we can refuse the prescriptions, all of this is left to the discretion of each individual in a liberal society, like smoking or drinking excessively. Second: You talk about normality, even preserving normality, but are you so sure you know what normality is, where pathological begins and normal ends in psychiatry? We all have in mind "crazy" people who consider themselves normal, people who have all the apparent signs of normality and who are actually "crazy", not to mention those precursors who were considered crazy by their time before being recognized later as geniuses.

To the first objection, I would respond with a figure that I believe undermines the idea of the omnipotence of freedom to counteract the harmful effects of the DSM. One would expect that this informed freedom, which must produce what is called in law an informed consent, would be exercised in such a sensitive area as parental responsibility, and that parents would look twice or even three times before agreeing to their offspring, whose brains are still developing, ingesting chemical substances whose long-term effects are still unknown. For example, the prescription of Ritalin[7] has increased fourfold in the last ten years in France.

Freedom of choice must be preserved, but it can only be exercised within a framework of honest information and communication and a diversity of comparative options. Unfortunately, this is not the case in psychiatry for many reasons, including the control of pharmaceutical laboratories over a large part of medical information and post-graduate training. They are, in a way, judge and jury. Some investigations even accuse them of falsifying studies or concealing results that go against their industrial and commercial aims.

In conclusion, the DSM, by multiplying the pathologies, by lowering the inclusion thresholds, by focusing almost exclusively on behaviours, by sticking only to a clinic

---

7. Ritalin is a psychostimulant prescribed for Attention Deficit Hyperactivity Disorder (ADHD) from the age of 6.

of observation and of the gaze, and not of listening, by refusing the context and the history of the subject as well as the different dimensions or structures, has not put an end to the ancestral fear of madness, nor has it advanced the delicate question of the segregation of the insane by one inch, but it has developed a factory of new mad people. False madmen, but who suffer for some of them the stigmatization with sometimes secondary benefits, as modest allowances of handicapped.

In the next chapter, I propose to try to answer the second objection, concerning normality, because it constitutes one of the prerequisites and criteria for judging the validity of a classification of mental illnesses. Moreover, we cannot decently denounce the DSM as a factory of madmen if we do not first have some criteria for differentiating the normal from the pathological in psychiatry. So can we answer the question: who is crazy and who is not?

2. Who is crazy, who is not?

The question of the norm in the field of psychiatry - which is now called mental health - has never been satisfactorily answered because of its complexity, and above all because each individual is unique in his or her way of being human, in his or her emotions, thoughts, moods, personality, but also in his or her reaction to medication, and especially to psychotropic drugs. Everyone can see this immediately and trivially: for example, the same dose of caffeine will not have the same effect on two individuals, one will fall asleep without difficulty, the other will suffer from insomnia.

More than elsewhere in medicine, the norm in psychiatry is also very difficult to define because certain psychiatric syndromes obviously have a cultural dimension which means that they are present in certain cultures and not in others, or present in a different form.

Is the psyche transcultural and universal?

The DSM, which claims to be universal in scope with the most objective descriptions possible, has in fact accentuated the difficulties of defining a norm. Because it is concerned specifically with behaviour, it is confronted with the fact that the norm for behaviour varies to varying degrees across cultures. For example, the social phobia described in the DSM is virtually non-existent in Japan, because the norm for social behaviour in Japan would be virtually the same as being a social phobic in the United States. This observation, which could fuel a certain cultural relativism, has divided the psychiatric community between certain ethno-psychiatrists who believe that the "phenotypes" of mental illnesses, i.e., the way in which these illnesses present themselves to the observer, are dependent on the culture and the language of expression, and certain theorists of transcultural psychiatry who assert, with regard to the main mental illnesses, that beyond the cultural variations, there are invariants that can be identified in all cultures.

For example, a "depressed person" labelled as such by the DSM in France will not necessarily be so in Iran, because the psychological suffering to which the depressive complaint testifies will be expressed differently, with, for example, in France, the importance of sleep disorders and, in Iran, the importance of somatic complaints.

But transcultural psychiatrists, while recognizing these differences, believe that there is a hard core, a common core of depression. Only part of the form of expression, the envelope, is modified. Only the formal framework of certain symptoms is dependent on the cultural and linguistic context. One could say, according to transcultural psychiatry, that mental pathologies are described in different ways according to the cultures but that there is a common definition.

The WHO has produced studies to compare the ways in which depression is expressed in different countries. For example, out of 100 patients labelled as depressed in Switzerland, 70% of them feel guilty, whereas only 38% in Iran. The same is true for suicidal ideation between Canadian and Japanese depressed patients, the difference is very significant. Is this just the appearance, the mask of depression, or do these variations call into question the very validity of the concept of depression? This question is important because if there is an invariant core to depression - and since depression is a pathology of mood one is entitled to think that there is some kind of universal norm for mood, which distinguishes between its "normal" variations, such as sadness, and the pathological ones that manifest themselves in depression - one can conclude that the norm has an objective existence.

Two safeguards: normativity and neurosis

In France, until the 1990s, two theoretical currents dominated the psychiatric scene: the organodynamism of Henri Ey and psychoanalysis. These two theoretical bodies of thought each have their own conception of psychological or mental normality.

For Henri Ey's organodynamism, the norm is not defined outside the psyche. It is inscribed in what he calls architectonics, in other words the architecture or structuring of the psyche. The consequence of this internal place of the norm is that what is normal belongs to psychic causality and what is pathological, to organic causality. In simpler terms, for Henri Ey, when a behavior, an emotion, a thought... comes under psychology, one remains in the normal variations of the psyche. He calls this psychovariations. When these same thoughts, emotions, affects exceed a certain threshold, they are related to modifications of the brain, of the organic. We note that Henri Ey does not define what is normal or the norm in psychiatry, but that he specifies what determines the barrier between the normal and the pathological.

This theory of organodynamism was dominant in France for decades, but from the beginning it was contested by psychoanalysis. Freud, far from being uninterested in the question of the norm, thought that his discoveries about neuroses, and therefore about pathology, could shed light on normal psychological functioning. The norm in the statistical sense does not concern him; he uses the word "norm" in contrast with a pathological state: normal equals non-paranoid, for example. Normality can concern a given or specific psychic character, for example ambivalence, which is not presented in the same way in the obsessive neurotic and in the normal subject.

In Freud, there are also occurrences where normality is an ideal notion to reach, as for example to reconcile obsessive, erotic and narcissistic traits. The norm can also appear as a fiction, the normal self not existing whereas the pathological self is a reality. Very important finally, for Freud there is in any pathological state, even the most serious, a part of normality.

Freud also used the clinical categories of psychiatric nosography[8], in particular *neurosis* and *psychosis*. How did he conceive their relationship to normality? The concept that best answers this question is the concept of functional normality. The normal differs from the neurotic only in functionality and not in mechanisms nor in psychic contents, which are the same. The normal person finds a "more elegant" solution to his psychic conflicts, as we say of a mathematical demonstration, or a more stable, more harmonious solution.

Psychosis is not in the continuity of the normal for psychoanalysis, except perhaps for Melanie Klein, as I have already said. But psychosis has a function: delirium, for example, is qualified by Freud as an attempt at healing. The function of psychosis is opposed to the meaning of neurosis. This idea of the function of psychosis can be compared with an original notion of Georges Canguilhem, the notion of *normativity*.

Normativity represents the capacity of the organism to produce new norms in order to adapt to the demands of life, in the same way that illness is an option available to the organism to adapt to new norms of biological life. The

---

8. Nosography is the description of disorders and diseases.

2. Who is crazy, who is not?

paradoxes and the complexity of the questions concerning the norm in psychiatry are well perceived when the onset of a delirium can be conceived as a testimony of the normativity shown by the psyche of a subject; at the same time, one cannot ignore that this form of normativity is abnormal. Moreover, the search for new norms of psychic functioning, if it is individual, is not less linked to the social life. The individual, and especially his psychic life, is always in interaction with the others.

In conclusion of this overview of the theories that dominated French psychiatry in the 20th century, we can say that they kept the idea of norm as a reference, and that the fundamental concept on which they were based was neurosis.

The end of the neurosis, the beginning of the disorders...

The dismantling of neurosis into several categories by the DSM was presented as a simplification; but in reality it had multiple consequences. To say that ordinary neurosis is the norm allows one to emphasize the dimension of conflict, which is inherent to neurosis. To live in normality is to find the best answers to the external and internal conflicts that are present in the psychic life. From this point of view, to treat is to help the neurotic patient to find the best solutions, those which allow him to find his normativity, that is to say a better symptomatic balance. The signs of his discomfort, such as anguish and mood disorders, must be respected to a certain degree because they are evidence of his search for a new balance. They are the witnesses of the "normativity in action". However, in the DSM, there is no neurosis, no conflict, no normativity. There are only disorders to be corrected, with no other meaning than a deviation from the norm established by the consensus. The neurosis, if it was in continuity with the state of normality to the point of being confused with it, was in discontinuity with the psychoses. In the DSM, deprived of structural markers, there are no indicators of discontinuity between the normal and the pathological, but indicators of a quantitative type to include such and such a state in a disorder. Therefore, normality and pathology belong to the same spectrum.

On the other hand, with the disappearance of neurosis, the disorders that were grouped in this category are autonomous and there is a levelling effect, disorder for disorder. If structures such as neurosis and psychosis no longer exist, what is the difference between an anxiety disorder and a delusional disorder? They both designate, if not a madman, at least a sick person. Thus, we can see how in an almost mechanical way the erasure of the neurosis, and thus of the structural dimension, leads to the medicalization of psychic life.

It is sometimes objected that the suppression of neurosis corresponds to a sociological and anthropological evolution. We would have passed from the man of neurotic conflict of the Freudian era to the biological man of the post-modern era, who would no longer suffer from conflicts but from deficits. The neurosis and its feeling of guilt would have been replaced by the depression and its narcissistic disorders. It seems to me that this statement is not a causal explanation but rather an afterthought. For my part, I would retain another hypothesis. It seems to me that our liberal society has changed the context of psychiatric care by making the search for the meaning of the psychic symptoms that the subject complains about a waste of time. There is also a refusal of exhaustiveness, a positioning on the regulation of behaviors, the correction of dysfunctions, the affirmation of the subject's autonomy and the refusal of alienation in the transference, assimilated to a position of dependence. In other words, everything that interferes with this sacrosanct autonomy of the subject - without exception - must be corrected. The DSM allows for self-diagnosis and gives the user a place as an expert who can discuss as an equal with the mental health professional. The DSM creates new patients, new madmen, who are experts on their illnesses!

I will evoke, or rather hazard another hypothesis to try to explain the continuous extension of the field of mental pathology with the concomitant reduction of the field of normality in the DSM. What contributes considerably to provoke "disorders" in social relations, to remain rebellious to education, to good morals, to social conventions? Sexual impulses, obviously. Let us take the example of dreams. Look at the dreamer who is alone, sheltered from his sleep, whose conscience has been relaxed and with it the requirements of life in society; how does he present himself? With many "disorders": he is aggressive, sometimes violent, panic-stricken, always deeply egoistic, murderous or incestuous on occasion, megalomaniac, etc., because he no longer controls his impulses. This makes me think that many of the disorders that the DSM talks about are in fact caused by the impulses. However, it only describes specific sexual disorders, eliminating the term sexual perversions and replacing it with the more sanitized and politically correct term *paraphilia*. If my hypothesis is correct, the hunt for disorders may turn out to be in some cases a hunt for impulses. Since drives accompany all aspects of life, if we want to reach the level of "zero drives", we must broaden the scope of the notion of disorders and lower the threshold at which we decide that there is a drive. The promoters of the DSM obviously do not have the objective that I assign to them, but this is happening without their knowledge.

In conclusion, I would say that whatever the many difficulties in determining who is crazy and who is not, who has a mental disorder and who does not, difficulties that I have tried to expose, it is appropriate to keep common sense. Shyness is not a social phobia, a child's agitation and concentration difficulties are rarely an attention deficit hyperactivity disorder, a sadness or a bereavement, even if intense, is not a major depressive state, an adolescent crisis is not a pathology, a sweet tooth is not an addiction, an isolated abuse of substances is not an addictive behaviour, tantrums in a young child are not the beginning of a disease, etc. If we do not keep this dividing line, the whole of existence becomes pathology.

3. Did you say hyperactive?

I was made aware of the thorny issue of chemical treatment of hyperactivity in children many years ago, when parents in open conflict with their 6 year old son came to consult me. I diagnosed a neurotic state in the child and motor and impulsive reactions not unrelated to the parents' anxieties. The treatment went well, the child's agitation was resolved and the parents showed, at least in appearance, a remarkable degree of cooperation. Until the moment when a television program, which I did not see, explained, it seems, from what the parents remembered, that there was now an appropriate remedy for certain child agitation syndromes that French child psychiatrists refused to prescribe out of psychoanalytical dogmatism. The impact of this program on the parents of the child I was following was very important. They stopped the treatment and went to a hospital service in order to have the drug in question prescribed to their child. They did not heed my warnings: the risk that this treatment would cause brain damage was proven. Fortunately, the prescription was a failure and they came back to consult.

Since this event, the prescription of Ritalin has increased in a rather worrying way. To try to understand the ins and outs of such an "epidemic", here is a clinical episode that is totally invented, but any resemblance with real situations is likely.

From DSM to child psychiatrist: Does ADHD exist?

This is the story of a family that everyone could relate to. The "hero" is named Eric. He is 6 years old and has always been unruly according to his parents. When asked for details, they explain that he doesn't sit still easily, often interrupts conversation, tries to get the adults' attention, often moves from one activity to another with impulsive gestures, loses his temper too often and, from their point of view, has become "unbearable" for some time. They can't take it anymore: Eric doesn't realize that he's not alone, that there's his little sister, that she exists too. Eric's parents ask for help because they are worried. The father is afraid of becoming violent; he feels the impulse to hit his son. He feels guilty about it. She described the boy's behaviour in class: he doesn't listen, he is distracted, he doesn't finish tasks except what interests him, he makes careless mistakes, he doesn't tidy up his things, she had to change his seat because he was heckling with his neighbor. One day, when she was reprimanding him, he answered "that he was tired of being argued with, that it was always his fault and that he was going to kill himself". She did not want to attach too much importance to Eric's words in order not to dramatize them, but she explained to his parents that if he persisted in his behavior, he would not be able to read by the end of the school year, and she alerted them to the risks of a bad start in school. But if she wanted to meet his parents, it was mainly because of a particular incident: during an outing, Eric seems to have caused a moment of distraction among the adults accompanying him, leading to a lack of supervision and the loss of sight of some children for a sufficiently long time to induce a state of panic in the teacher in charge of the outing. After this episode, she perceived a significant exacerbation of Eric's problems and, reluctantly, thought that he was becoming a danger to the group, that he had exceeded the tolerance threshold and that his case was pathological. Yet Eric had been purposely placed in her class because he had already been "screened", or rather identified, in kindergarten. The teachers had met to discuss his case and had thought that this teacher was the best person to deal with Eric, as Mrs. B. is known for her calmness, tolerance and flexibility. When Mrs. B revealed to her colleagues that she could no longer tolerate Eric's behavior, the image of the child changed in the minds of the teachers and the principal: "If even Mrs. B can't do anything with Eric, he is really sick.

3. Did you say hyperactive?

From this interview with Mrs. B., Eric's parents came out of it anxious despite the precautions that Eric's teacher took to "put the situation into perspective". They looked at all the elements that are negative indicators for Eric's school future, in particular the statistics that can be consulted on the Internet, which "demonstrate" that failure in the preparatory course is often a bad prognosis.

The teacher advised a consultation with a psychologist or a medical-psychological-pedagogical center (CMPP) and spoke to them about Ritalin, while refusing to give an indication instead of the child psychiatrist. She did her job, she spoke to the parents from the start of the "serious" schooling, she did not accuse them or even implicate them in Eric's disorders. She merely tried to prevent what she saw as a dangerous development. Eric's parents, on the other hand, had asked about Ritalin and were rather dubious, even against this prescription. But if the child psychiatrist considers it appropriate, they may change their minds.

Faced with a situation like that of Eric and his parents, one can imagine several possible outcomes. For my part, I will imagine three different ones.

First, the most plausible version today: Eric's father talks about his son's difficulties to Eric's grandfather, who is a rheumatologist and who advises him to consult a professor of child psychiatry who is not a psychoanalyst. Indeed, he thinks, given what he knows and what he hears from Eric's father, that his grandson suffers from Attention Deficit Hyperkinesia Disorder (ADHD), that this syndrome is linked to a cerebral dysfunction that cannot be fixed by psychoanalysis, and that it must be treated with Ritalin. He read in a medical journal that this disorder was more and more frequent, that it was now possible to detect it. He advises Eric not to consult the CMPP closest to his home because he knows that precious time will be wasted and that Eric's parents will be asked a lot of intrusive questions that have nothing to do with the child's disorder. Eric's parents took this "informed" advice and went to a "state-of-the-art" hospital with their son. Eric underwent a battery of tests, the parents were questioned conscientiously, but only about Eric's medical history: how the pregnancy had gone, intercurrent infections, family history and Eric's behaviour. There were no specific questions about Eric's interaction with his parents, other than formal yes/no questions. They were offered an appointment in one month with a possible period of day hospitalization to refine the diagnosis and decide on the course of action. The parents are satisfied, reassured by the serious context of high scientific technicality. They trust professionals in white coats.

Curiously, during the two weeks following the consultation, Eric was much calmer, as the teacher had also noticed. The improvement in Eric's behavior would almost have the effect of encouraging the parents to give up any therapeutic approach, but they do not dare take this risk and feel committed to the hospital. When they return, they will receive a diagnosis and treatment after a new series of tests. The diagnosis is what the grandfather had imagined: attention deficit disorder with hyperkinesia. The treatment is Ritalin, five days a week and only during school periods. They were informed of the possible side effects, and after two appointments devoted to adjusting the doses of Ritalin - because Eric was experiencing insomnia, a known side effect at the beginning of treatment - a new consultation was scheduled within six months. Eric's parents went online again and found that they were not alone in their difficulties. They participate in forums, exchange ideas on what to do. But Eric has a label: he has a mental illness, or at least a syndrome that handicaps him, and the parents, outside of the forums, don't really feel supported, especially by the health care team, as appointments are on the dotted line.

Now, let's leave the world of fiction for a moment to think about the possible consequences of this medicalized and scientific approach to Eric's problems. On the face of it, everything has been done according to the proper medical method: exploration, evaluation, diagnosis and treatment. But in reality, I will explain why this medical approach is akin to pretending. Eric is going to receive a molecule at the age of 6; this molecule is an amphetamine derivative likely to cause growth retardation, cardiac problems, and whose long-term effects are not clearly established. It is therefore appropriate to at least ask whether Eric is really sick, or sick to the point of receiving this treatment which is not harmless.

First of all, according to the DSM-4, Eric shows signs that are classifiable as ADHD, but also in other categories such as depression and even oppositional defiant disorder. He doesn't fit neatly into one category, which is common for children this age with these types of disorders. It's called comorbidity, which means having more than one disorder at the same time. But this does not dispel the confusion, quite the contrary. With Eric's case, we are faced with the major question posed by ADHD: is it a syndrome with validity or is it a grouping of signs and behaviors left to the subjective appreciation of the clinical observer or the child's entourage?

My answer is clear: in the form described in the DSM-4, ADHD is a chimera with blurred contours encompassing truly hyperactive children, long known to psychiatry, and children whose motor skills and attention do not exceed, or barely exceed, variations of normal, not to mention changes due to reactions to life events that may persist in interaction with adults. ADHD in the DSM is an "imaginary disease" which has resulted in an explosion in the prescription of Ritalin. The prescription of Ritalin tripled in France between 2000 and 2005[9]. The defenders of the DSM version of ADHD point to studies showing that ADHD children are more likely than others to become delinquents and to have addictions to psychoactive substances. It seems to me somewhat paradoxical to claim to fight against future addictions by administering an amphetamine derivative classified as a narcotic drug to a child for an indefinite period of time.

There is no question of considering that ADHD was created only to market Ritalin, although there are convergences and conflicts of interest between psychiatrists, pharmaceutical companies and some others. But the simple fact that it is included in the classification,

---

9. Prieur (Cécile), "Des enfants sages sur ordonnance", *Le Monde*, 23 November 2005.

3. Did you say hyperactive?

it becomes a real disease. It exists and then there is a knock-on effect that pushes for its detection, which in turn validates its reality.

But if Eric doesn't get a prescription for Ritalin, what should be done to ease the situation?

Here is the second version of this fictional story. Eric's parents go to the CMPP where they are seen by a clinical psychologist and psychoanalyst. At first, the interview takes place in the presence of Eric and his two parents. Eric was then seen alone and, finally, it was the parents' turn to be seen without their son. A few key points emerged: Eric had not been able to cope at all with the birth of his little sister; he had learned that his parents had "lost" a baby to sudden death before he was born, and the words "lost", "losing", "loss" were often used in the parents' comments and in Eric's recent history. For example, Eric overreacted when he felt accused by the teacher of having caused some of the children in the group to "lose" their sight on the famous field trip. Eric talks about his nightmares about being lost in the woods, etc.

Eric agrees to come back for a consultation on the condition that his parents come back too. He was offered interviews with the psychologist and participation in a group, led by another psychologist in the company of a psychomotrician. Thanks to a collage workshop, Eric will experiment with his ability to dream and act alone in the presence of others. The psychologist who follows Eric also sees the parents on a regular basis. After several consultations, Eric's parents did not receive a diagnosis from the CMPP. They did not know exactly what was going on during the interviews, nor during the workshop sessions. They understand that Eric has a "defect in the ability to use the imagination, which hinders his ability to think," but this doesn't mean anything to them. They were simply told that Eric felt like an outsider in his class, that he had been demonized by the school. But now that Eric is being monitored, the teacher feels reassured. The "team" had informed the school that Eric was not crazy, that he was overreacting, but that talking, restraint, and the mediation of collage would help him. Eric's parents felt supported, but the lack of a diagnosis, of understandable reference points, was somewhat disorienting. If things don't get better, they may lose patience.

In both versions of my story, I can envisage a favorable or unfavorable outcome. But I prefer to imagine a third version in which Eric is seen by a child psychiatrist, or a clinical psychologist, who will evaluate according to clinical criteria, and not those of the DSM, Eric's global situation: the interaction of his disorders with his parents, his history. He will listen to Eric and not just observe him with neutrality. He will explain to the parents that if he does not calm down quickly, medication will have to be considered, but that Ritalin does not cure him, only prevents behaviours that lead to handicaps, in particular learning delays. He added that Ritalin was not enough, that it was imperative to provide other therapeutic treatment for the child as well as support for the parents - sometimes called guidance - because Eric's disorder was also relational, and its etiology was not known.

The child psychiatrist or psychologist was cautious about using medication, but his training in psychopatho-

3. Did you say hyperactive?

logy and his clinical experience enabled him to identify a large number of defense mechanisms in Eric that were similar to neurosis. Her in-depth interviews with the parents succeeded in bringing to light the particular and very conflicting place that Eric occupied in their history as a couple, their projections onto Eric unknowingly maintaining the situation. Eric escaped the unnecessary prescription of Ritalin and the stigma of a psychiatric diagnosis. His appeasement will not be the consequence of a chemical action on the brain, but the effect of modifications in the family's psychic economy, and will be all the more stable. The parents will have the opportunity to express their feelings of guilt about Eric, but they will not be made to feel guilty in any way. Their involvement in their son's problems is related to their role as responsible educators of their child.

How to invent a disorder from symptoms

So much for our three scenarios, which seem to me to overlap with many real-life family stories. What can we say, based on this example, that will allow the reader to better understand the health issues? With regard to ADHD, the DSM inevitably leads those who use it as a diagnostic tool to overdiagnose or misdiagnose, because it takes as an unproven implicit idea that the disorder is related to a minor brain lesion or brain dysfunction, as if it were something objective or objectifiable. This is not the case. ADHD is a grouping of symptoms that have in common that they are sensitive to certain medications and that the DSM has constituted as a disorder that manifests itself largely in social interaction. Its "functional" impact depends on the environment, its level of tolerance, its responses; as a result, the criteria for inclusion in ADHD are not objective. It is almost necessary to reverse the terms of observation and dare to say that, in some cases, the disorder in question is the disorder that the child causes to his environment, hence the key idea that this disorder must be corrected as soon as possible. However, the disorder that a child causes is a very vague and delicate concept that depends on multiple factors, especially social factors. An anxious child with a tendency to react repeatedly with agitation to certain situations or contexts is much more likely to be labelled ADHD by the average practitioner using the DSM if he or she comes from a disadvantaged background, with educational inconsistencies and cramped housing, than if he or she belongs to an affluent social environment, with comfortable housing conditions. This is a far cry from scientific objectivity.

The "old" psychiatric clinic tried to distinguish schematically between hyperkinesia belonging to a serious pathology, true hyperkinesia, and behaviours, reactions of agitation in a neurotic context. With this framework of thought, only truly hyperkinetic children, or those for whom appeasement cannot be obtained by any other means, in particular educational and psychotherapeutic (dynamic psychotherapy, behaviorist or psychodrama), are eligible for Ritalin prescription. Beyond the difference in approach between the clinic and the DSM, there is an epistemological difference that can be stated as follows:

are agitation, fluctuations in concentration, and impulsivity in a child above a certain threshold only disorders to be corrected or eradicated like a toothache, or are they also symptoms that carry a meaning? Why is Ritalin so successful that it is, as I said, considered a miracle drug even though it is not curative?

The risk of disempowerment

Ritalin allows for rapid sedation of the disorder and allows for the idea that parents are not responsible, which is true; but they are still in a position of responsibility as parents. Giving Ritalin to a neurotic child with ADHD-like disorders can be a miracle for parents who tend to give up. But the sedation of the disorder without any psychic elaboration on their part risks confirming them in their attitude of resignation, the pleasure principle that regulates our psychic functioning consisting in wanting to obtain the appeasement of tensions at the lowest cost. It is not only the pharmaceutical laboratories that are indirectly pushing for the inflation of the diagnosis of ADHD, but also the evolution of society, as they say, with the extension of the application of the pleasure principle in all places where children live, family, school, various institutions. However, ADHD defeats this pleasure principle, hence the rejection of these children, their demonization, as in Eric's example. The traditional approach was not without disadvantages, in particular that of wrongly accrediting the idea of parental guilt or of allowing the disturbing situation to evolve for too long, in the expectation of a hoped-for appeasement, or of a modification of the family's psychic economy whose agitation revealed its pathological nature.

In conclusion, on ADHD and the DSM, I would say that the major risks are above all the inflation of the diagnosis, the imprudent and extensive prescription due to a political tendency more and more asserted in psychiatry to correct behaviors without taking the time to stop on the always singular meaning for each child of these behaviors. On the other hand, we know that the education of children is problematic, that teachers are often confronted with difficult situations, and that in many cases diagnosed as ADHD, it is not only a matter of lowering the tolerance threshold of adults, but also of educational deficiencies and social problems, so that we can ask ourselves: is Ritalin the new opium of the "parental people"?

4. Depression for all

Depression, which in common parlance is called a nervous breakdown, is a relatively new disease, which has existed for only a little over half a century. It is true that melancholy has been described and studied since the dawn of time, and that it has given rise to magnificent pictorial representations by Dürer or Munch, to mention only the most famous, but the concept of depression, a medical concept, is recent.

Depression represents a typical example of what I have called the factory of the insane. It is paradigmatic of the trend towards diagnostic inflation and concentrates a large number of factors that have led psychiatry to move towards excessive medicalization.

Depression appears as a kind of final common path between normal reactions to life's accidents, on the one hand, such as bereavements, break-ups, failures, illnesses, harassment at work, etc. - what we call the tragic dimension of existence - and, on the other hand, as the real pathologies of mood, the authentic depressive syndromes. - What we call the tragic dimension of existence - and, on the other hand, as the real pathologies of the mood, the authentic depressive syndromes. The confusion between these phenomena, which should not be subsumed under the same category, reaches a peak with the DSM-5, particularly with the example of bereavement already given above.

A pathology built from drugs?

Psychiatry has constructed depression as a pathological state essentially under the impact of antidepressants, which have proved effective and, in the process, have redrawn the contours of the syndromes. For example, the classic endogenous (psychotic, unipolar or bipolar depression) and exogenous (symptomatic depression such as neurosis or psychosis) distinction has disappeared from the DSM. All depressions are now on the same level and automatically treated with antidepressants. However, the old category of exogenous depression, which contains what is also called neurotic depression, has not become invalid - to the point that some recommend its return to the DSM - and, above all, it constitutes the vast majority of depressions seen by the general practitioner. This fact has prompted the health authorities to conduct information campaigns, sometimes with the help of pharmaceutical laboratories, among general practitioners, who were only able to detect 20% of depressive states. From this point of view, the DSM provides considerable help by serving as a model for formalized interviews that allow rapid diagnoses, thanks to which new depressed patients are recruited and prescribed antidepressants. For the laboratories, it is an expansion of the market, and for the patients, it is a help that alleviates their symptoms and allows them to associate them with an illness and not with psychological conflicts. This can lead to a reduction in guilt but also to a reduction in responsibility.

As antidepressants became more effective, their simplified handling led to an increase in their prescription. Almost all depressives have been lumped into the catch-all category of bipolar, a category that is entirely drug-related. But we are all bipolar. For example, our moods vary throughout the day: we may feel a little sad in the morning, then more cheerful during the day until an upset darkens our thoughts, and finally, in the evening, be in a good mood again and even a little elated. The same cycle, with some modifications, will repeat itself the following days. If the mood worsens in one direction or the other, we enter the field of pathology. There would be a mood cycle as there is a sleep/wake cycle, a biological cycle whose disturbances, designated as disorders, should be corrected by antidepressant or mood regulating drugs. But this alleged biological cycle has not received any scientific proof, no validation by science; but it speaks to the "scientific imagination", it is a satisfactory construction for the mind and it is an argument of medical-commercial rhetoric.

In the 1950s and 1960s, the image of depression was linked to stars, to celebrities whose suicide attempts made headlines. But with the development and diffusion of antidepressants, it has been "democratized". Depression continues to interest media professionals, those who "make the opinion". It regularly makes the front page of certain magazines where they warn against hidden depression, latent depression or unrecognized depression. Beware of those who are depressed but who deny it, refuse it or ignore it: it is dangerous and we call on those around us because the refusal to admit the illness or the lack of energy to decide to treat oneself are part of the pathology. Anybody can fall into depression, the risk is generalized because of the living conditions, and we advise people to go and see a doctor as soon as the first signs appear, such as insomnia, a feeling of emptiness, moral weariness. What the public does not know is that this "illness" is entirely constructed under the influence of antidepressant drugs, which makes me say that if biological psychiatry initially constructed depression, depression contributes to constructing biological psychiatry in return. It serves as its paragon, it is its emblem.

We are facing an epidemic of depression in all Western societies. In France, the number of cases of depression has increased eightfold from 1970 to 2010. Children are also affected by depression. Until now, they have escaped the prescription of antidepressants, as most of these products have not obtained the marketing authorization (MA) for people under 16 years old, at least in France. The WHO considers the fight against depression to be one of the main causes of public health worldwide and this epidemic would be the mark of the success of biological psychiatry, known as "scientific", which has taken precedence over the old doctrines that are now outdated, first and foremost psychoanalysis, which is based on the idea of conflict, which would be replaced, according to Ehrenberg, by the "fatigue of being oneself".

Is there any scientific basis for depression?

It can be said that at the present time biological psychiatry has totally failed in its attempt to scientifically found psychiatry. Psychiatric diagnosis remains entirely clinical, and the etiology of mental illnesses awaits explanation. At the same time, there is an incredible dynamism in the pharmaceutical industry, with new psychotropic drugs being marketed on a regular basis, even though there are no biological markers for these different disorders. Usually, the research of the effectiveness of a new drug on a disease is done through several phases of clinical trials, the first of which is carried out on cells, tissues or on animals. In general, there is a reliable control corresponding to the disease, for example a virus or a bacterium. If a drug is to be tested, the causal agent, known as a "reliable control", is injected into the animal in order to evaluate the effectiveness of the drug. In the field of mental illness, there is no reliable control because the etiology is unknown. Nevertheless, new drugs are tested on animals; it is not a question of making a mouse depressed, but of trying to reproduce and compare the effects induced by the drug with the effects produced by antidepressants in humans. This is an empirical method of pharmaco-induction, but it is very successful from the point of view of drug research, which is why new molecules are flooding the market.

Thus, there is a confusion between the dynamism of the research, which is sustained, and its real scientific advances, which are non-existent or almost non-existent. This way of proceeding, particular to psychiatric pharmacological research, allows to detail one by one the behaviours and one by one the emotions on which the products act. The result is an exclusive interest in a psychiatry of observable behavior, of immediate and purely conscious emotions. This is precisely what the DSM offers, with two consequences: a synergy between pharmacological research and the evolution of the DSM nosographic categories, and an ever-increasing pathologization of emotions and behaviours in response to the expanded scope of psychotropic drugs. There is no need to mention conflicts of interest or any conspiracy: a simple knock-on effect is sufficient to explain this synergy.

There is also another explanation for this concordance between the DSM and the pharmaceutical industry; it is what Lacan would perhaps have called "the push-to-science[10]", that is to say the illusion of a scientific

---

10. I owe this explanation to Dr. Bernard Odier, head of the policlinic of the Association de santé mentale du XIIIe arrondissement (ASM13).

understanding of the mechanisms of depression in humans, since antidepressants act and we can identify with increasing precision their mode of action on neuro-mediators. The desire to consider that the etiology of depression is known, or even that it is within reach, has pushed psychiatrists into the dead ends of reductionism and into naturalistic errors. The brainless psychiatry of the psychoanalysts has been replaced by a psychiatry without psyche, a psychiatry of the "mental body" according to the happy expression of Pignarre.

For a reasoned prescription of antidepressants

But this evolution of psychiatry has also given rise to a lot of resistance. More and more voices in the United States and in Europe are being raised against the trivialization and generalization of the prescription of antidepressants, which are not harmless drugs (they have cardiovascular consequences, for example). First of all, I quote Professor David Healy who denounces, with evidence and studies to back it up, the harmfulness of the wrong prescription of antidepressants. It is difficult, if not impossible, to measure the percentage of patients on antidepressants who are treated wrongly or for too long with these products, but, according to my own practice, it is a significant proportion.

We need to return to a reasonable posture. Not everyone who is labelled depressed by the DSM criteria or their equivalents is ill, and not everyone who is ill should be treated with antidepressants. The ability to get depressed is part of the psyche's defense mechanism to elaborate certain situations, to adapt to certain changes; and, in some cases, the short-circuiting imposed by antidepressants by abrading this defense mechanism can be harmful. A comparison with the over-prescription of anti-biotics, which weakens the immune system, could be taken as a rough image. Some people have found a word to designate this positivity of depression, Professor Pierre Fédida in particular: it is *depressivity*[11]. Depressivity is animation, vital impetus, whereas depression is on the side of the inanimate. Depressivity can be used as an alternative because it requires talking with the patient, listening to him or her in order to evaluate the extent to which his or her vital momentum has been affected by the situation. This depression will be the motor of his restart, of his psychic reanimation and of his recovery. Clinically, the depressive symptoms can be very intense but if the depression can be mobilized, then the prescription of antidepressants will be useless or will possibly have a simple role of accompaniment to attenuate anguish and inhibition in order to protect a space of speech: it is a question of the patient talking about what is happening to him, of putting the episode he is going through in the context of his life, of giving it a place or a function.

The untimely, isolated and reckless prescription of antidepressants weakens the possibilities of recourse to depression, sometimes giving the feeling of having

---

11. Fédida (Pierre), *Des bienfaits de la dépression. Éloge de la psycho-thérapie*, Paris, Odile Jacob, coll. "Poches Odile Jacob", 2003.

been artificially brought out of depression, only thanks to medication, and of not having been listened to. This is in serious contrast to the image often broadcast in the media of effective psychotropic drugs and endless analytical psychotherapy. The best way to space out depressive episodes, or even prevent them, is to allow the patient to use his or her psychic abilities.

In true bipolar disorder, such as the former manic-depressive psychosis, the problem is different. In this case, it is advocated that the patient's ability to detect the warning signs of a relapse should be strengthened at an early stage, with the aim of prevention. This therapeutic approach is debatably called psycho-education. It is also important to help the patient to accept this "disease" that has come upon him or her.

In conclusion, I want to emphasize that the psychiatrist's job should be to refuse a stereotyped response in all cases, to consider that not all depressive moments that the patient goes through are pathological, because some crisis phenomena, critical moments of existence, are part of normality. It is not enough to identify the symptoms of depression with the help of the DSM. It is also necessary to take into account the facts of psychopathological observation which, contrary to what some people claim, are not in the realm of speculation: a depression will not have the same consequences and will not produce the same reorganizations in a neurotic and in a psychotic. In the case of depression, psychiatry, under the influence of the DSM, has gone much too far down the road of "a-clinical". This has resulted in over-diagnosis, over-prescription of psychotropic drugs and an excessive reorientation towards a social vocation of rehabilitation, reintegration and over-protection, all of which end up being harmful in the long run to the objective it has set itself, namely the mental health of the patient. The more depressives are "manufactured", the less well they are treated.

A return to a certain transversality of concepts (pharmacology, psychopathology) is desirable. The possible plurality of approaches to depression is an opportunity. It is necessary in the interest of patients and corresponds better to the difficult but nevertheless accessible objective of reconciling psychological complexities with therapeutic effectiveness.

5. The new DSM has arrived

An event has occurred in the world of psychiatry: the publication of version 5 of the DSM. Let's extract some ideas from it, suitable to illustrate my thesis of the factory of the insane.

How to persuade someone that they have a medical condition

I imagine an individual who recently celebrated his sixtieth birthday, who has no psychiatric antecedents, who has no neurological illnesses, who is not taking any psychotropic drugs; if he cannot regularly remember certain names or words, if he looks for his belongings, his keys for example, more often than in the past, if he is obliged to write down things so as not to forget, but if he keeps his head, he will be rightly inclined to attribute his memory difficulties to his age. His problems are minor and he remembers that his mother had the same problems at his age. It doesn't occur to him that what is happening to his memory is very different from what happened to his eyesight nearly twenty years ago when his ophthalmologist told him he had midlife presbyopia. So he simply has the somewhat painful feeling that the years are passing and that he has to live with it. But our man has a dream, or rather a nightmare, in which his aunt, his father's sister who died a few years ago, had Alzheimer's. He remembers the trauma he had when he visited her one day and she did not recognize him. After this dream, a little destabilized, he goes to consult a psychiatrist to be reassured. If the psychiatrist is "up to date", if he is informed of the content of the DSM-5, then our man will be diagnosed with minor cognitive disorders. When he asks, because of the hereditary factor, if these disorders are related to the onset of a dementia, he receives an evasive answer. The psychiatrist advises him to undergo a battery of tests to rule out the possibility of dementia and is careful to point out that there is no appropriate treatment for minor cognitive impairment.

Our man has become a patient, he has entered the field of pathology thanks to the psychiatric discourse of the DSM. In the days following the consultation, his memory problems worsen, his anxiety increases, which in turn reflects on the disorders, to the point that we no longer know which is first, the "minor cognitive disorder" or the anxiety. His wife rightly points out a paradox: he went to see a specialist because he was worried, and he came out of the consultation even more worried. But she is hopeful that everything will go back to normal as soon as he takes his tests: the tests are scientific and objective.

Unfortunately, he only gets an appointment in three months because there are few specialized centers with neuropsychologists who are qualified to perform this type of testing and, above all, it seems that an epidemic of minor cognitive disorders has just broken out, which is saturating the already limited capacity of these centers.

While waiting for the consultation, our patient's anxiety becomes very distressing. He then goes to see his general practitioner who prescribes a benzodiazepine, recommending that he take it as little as possible. But after a few days, the patient has the impression that he is losing his memory even more. He goes to the drug's package insert, where memory problems are listed as a side effect, and completes his information on the Internet. On the web, he learns that the prescription of benzodiazepines is associated with an increased risk of dementia after a certain age. Even before finishing the reading that would have shown him that he was not really concerned by this risk, he panics. He decided to stop taking the benzodiazepine, which led to several difficult nights with unusual insomnia.

After a few days, he has another moment of panic at the thought that he is exhausted and will not be able to meet his obligations, that he will lose his job and that, being a few years away from retirement, he will not find anything or be able to claim his rights. His mood darkens. His family and friends are worried, but he does not want to go back to see the psychiatrist who diagnosed him with his "illness" or the general practitioner who prescribed the anxiolytic. He nevertheless agrees to see another general practitioner who is recommended to him.

He makes an appointment with Dr. N., who has just been informed by a laboratory representative of the existence of a drug presented, with "scientific proof, curves and figures on glossy paper", as being very effective both in panic disorders and in depressive states. This representative left Dr. N. with a *guideline for* detecting a depressive state with a few questions. Before leaving, this representative made a point of specifying that, very often, depression was masked, that comorbidity with the disorders was frightening, that a generalized anxiety disorder was frequent, and that the "experts" of the DSM-5 had wondered about including an anxiety-depressive disorder in the new edition.

Our man will leave the consultation with a diagnosis of comorbidity (panic disorder and major depressive episode) and a prescription for an antidepressant (the molecule in question is an antidepressant). I'll let you imagine the rest, but let me ironically conclude this fiction and say to this patient: "Welcome to the club, not of the depressed, but of those who consume antidepressants!"

Is gluttony a mental disorder?

The DSM-5 has other surprises in store for us. Let's change the context and imagine a young woman, Ms. T., who is in her thirties and has a partner. They are planning to get married next fall and are thinking of having a child. She has a stable professional activity and she finds interest in her work. She has somehow "inherited" from her family, and in particular from her parents, a habit of eating a little too much in certain circumstances, festive or not. For her parents, cooking is an important value; they both come from regions renowned for their gastronomy and regularly cook hearty meals.

One night while indulging in her sweet tooth at a delicious dinner party, a guest mentions what he learned on the Internet: 12 binge eating episodes in three months is binge *eating disorder.* "It's a mental disorder," he says. Everyone starts laughing and calling each other binge eaters. Ms. T. laughs too. But she feels embarrassed and "confused" by what the guest is saying. She feels ashamed about her eating behaviour. Little by little, the idea creeps into her mind that what seemed to be a legitimate pleasure is wrong. She tries to count the number of times she has had bouts of gluttony, but cannot. She tries again to count, and finally concludes that she is within the scope of the diagnosis.

She sleeps poorly the next night, but she does not immediately relate this disturbance to what she has heard from the guest. She finds that memories of shameful moments from her childhood come back to her. She loses her appetite and refuses to go to restaurants several times,

5. The new DSM has arrived

which upsets her partner. She finally realizes that the diagnosis she verified at the party has affected her, but she wonders why.

Miss T... could, from this destabilization, turn to a psychoanalyst to try to know a little more, or sink into a phase of torment which can lead her to depression, or even overcome the affair by herself after a certain time. I leave all the hypotheses open without choosing or deciding, they are all plausible. What is important to me here is to show the effect of the announcement of a psychiatric diagnosis. Learning that one may be suffering from a mental disorder can have uncontrollable effects.

Miss T... found herself unconsciously in the position of someone who is caught in the act of solitary pleasure - her gluttony is an erotic type of pleasure -, and to hear that it is pathological causes her a feeling of shame. She feels as if she is stripped naked in public, which is enough to explain her persistent discomfort. But there's more. I said it, the parents of Miss T. are also greedy: this diagnosis resounds like a disavowal of a part of the family values, it modifies the glance which she has on this custom of the "banquets" and on her parents. The excess of food represented for Miss T... a way to receive the love of her parents. Good food is their preferred emotional expression, it is their way of giving. The DSM-5 diagnosis acted as a religious discourse prescribing a ban and affected her self-esteem. Miss T. entered a conflictual phase.

This case of diagnosis illustrates the fact that the DSM tracks down all our tendencies, all our pleasures in daily life, in order to pathologize them and correct them if necessary. It fulfils the function of a real bible that legislates what is allowed and what is forbidden.

Miss T... appears to be quite fragile to be destabilized to this extent; but psychologically fragile people must have all our consideration, in particular that of psychiatrists. On the other hand, we are all fragile because we all have areas of fragility: this is not synonymous with mental illness.

How the DSM stigmatizes young children

My last example concerns a new diagnosis, *disruptive mood disfunction disorder* (DMDD), which affects children between the ages of 6 and 18 who are having rage attacks. The word *disruptive* may be equivalent to the French word perturbant or perturbateur.

Following a report by the National Institute of Health and Medical Research (INSERM) in 2005, there was talk of a screening campaign for disruptive children in kindergarten. Then an attempt was made to screen for behavioral problems, again in kindergarten. Finally, in 2009-2010, the campaign to classify children at risk or at high risk. The DSM nosographic categories such as Oppositional Defiant Disorder or ADHD are vectors of this type of campaign, which are carried out in the name of prevention, but which are in reality operations to sort the wheat from the chaff, with incalculable consequences for children. A 6-year-old who has three or more disproportionate tantrums per week for several months may be diagnosed with DMMD. Of course,

5. The new DSM has arrived

there are precautions regarding age and the presence of other signs, but this diagnosis is likely to be over-represented. On the other hand, it is not validated by reliable studies, nor is it predictive of disorders in adulthood. It is a pure chimera produced by the malaise in parenting and education.

Previously, I have discussed the impact of the announcement effect of a psychiatric diagnosis. This is particularly true for children, as the diagnosis can lead to stigmatization and damage to the self-image of a developing psyche. Children are among the most vulnerable in society. An angry child, in my experience, often calls for "concern for him". This is implicitly recognized by the "inventors" of DMMD, who noted its greater prevalence in contexts of educational deficiency or inconsistency.

Is the choice to have the child carry a diagnostic label helpful to care? Yes, if only medication is considered, otherwise it is counterproductive. Taking into account the suffering of the child and his entourage, the impasse that led to the symptom, would be much wiser and more useful for treating the child. There is a great difficulty in general in child psychiatry: to take into account the variations that remain in the normal and that concern a developing subject and the reversibility, as well as the emotionality, of the disorders. Every child psychiatrist must keep these variations in mind. Moreover, in the case of these disorders affecting the child, the diagnosis being based on subjective appreciations emanating from the persons involved, redoubled caution is required to differentiate between variations of the normal and the pathology.

The major problem with these DSM diagnostic categories (DMMD, ADHD, etc.) as they apply to children is also that they are implicitly fixated. They function as labels that have the disadvantage of petrifying suffering and whose evolution is conceived essentially in terms of future risks, with the underlying idea of disability. It is recommended to detect the latter as early as possible, which prompts health and political authorities to promote campaigns starting from kindergarten. But this is a broad concept of disability, encompassing not only instrumental functions such as language or motor skills, but also living in a community, which does not lend itself to a simple objective evaluation, because it is not always independent of the child's family history and the social environment in which he or she grows up. If the child feels rejected or is unable to object through ordinary channels, he or she will be more prone to temper tantrums. It is known that in some American states, a child is ten times more likely to be labelled with Oppositional Defiant Disorder, ADHD, and sometimes DMMD, if he or she is black and from a disadvantaged background than if he or she is white and from an affluent background.

This observation should make us think and ask again about the nature of this "handicap". Is it biological, psychological or social? By intellectual ease, some psychiatrists answer: all three, hence an aggravation of the confusion of roles and responsibilities within child professionals. Fixism, i.e., the implicit adherence to the idea that there is no transformation or mutation within the diagnostic categories, is inadmissible; moreover, since it has no scientific basis, it is at the origin of the questionable social constructions that are certain disorders, and it tends to reverberate throughout the architecture of the classification: for example, in the DSM-5, a person who uses an illicit substance for the first time, or who commits his or her first abuse, is grouped with regular users in the name of risk. But how can we not see in this grouping a fixist ideology which goes against clinical evidence and therapeutic conduct? The abuse of a substance, just once, by an adolescent can have an initiatory value, a risk-taking value, to prove to himself that he has left the over-protected world of childhood and to assert his opposition to the law of adults, etc. Of course, this act must be taken seriously, but in no case automatically equated with an entry into addiction.

In conclusion, it is perhaps appropriate to qualify my assessment of the DSM: it does not only produce mad people, it also produces handicapped people, and the fight against the single thought of the DSM is a fight against fixist theories.

6. Can psychiatric diagnosis be scientific?

How is a diagnosis made in psychiatry? If the method based on the DSM is not the right one, if there are no biological markers or radiological images that can guide the diagnostic process, if there is a tendency to over-diagnose - what I call manufacturing madmen -, what is the right rule of diagnostic art in psychiatry?

The perceptual phenomenon

The clinical approach, in a way traditional, consists of having an interview with the patient, talking with him, asking him questions about his complaint, listening to him, receiving him, and taking into account the effects of his presence and his words on the clinician.

With such a system, which decides to dispense with more objective assessment instruments such as tests or formalized interviews at the outset, one could imagine that the diagnostic process is totally arbitrary, that it does not respond to any law and that it is a mystery. In reality, old studies[12] have shown that the psychiatric diagnosis was very often made by the psychiatrist in the first few minutes of the interview, and that this early diagnosis was confirmed at the end of the investigation by the same clinician in three quarters of the cases. Moreover, the early diagnosis has a higher reliability than later diagnoses. In other words, there is more agreement between different clinicians for the same patient when these clinicians make an early diagnosis, which could be translated in common language as: it is a diagnosis that jumps out at observers. Conversely, the later it is, the more hesitant it is, and the less reliable it is.

So, what hypotheses can we put forward about the mechanisms of this diagnostic approach? Some have thought that the clinician is sensitive to a form, because a form is immediately recognizable, it does not require a recapitulative reasoning, an exhaustive and additive inventory. But what is this form? It is a perceptive phenomenon which does not necessarily touch the field of the known phenomena of psychiatric semiology.

---

12. See in particular GAURON (Eugene F.), DICKINSON (John K.), "Diagnostic Decision Making in Psychiatry, I. Information Usage," *Archives of General Psychiatry*, vol. 14, 1966, p. 225-232.

I am thinking in particular of the overall quality of the patient's presentation or of what he or she arouses in the clinician, in the clinician's experience. This form short-circuits the medical approach, which breaks down into three stages and which the DSM wants to transpose into psychiatry: first, the collection of data, i.e. the signs, then the comparison with typical symptomatic configurations known by the clinician or with the help of a classification, and finally, the therapeutic decision, what is called the course of action, which is made by inference from the results of this comparison.

How to recognize schizophrenia: the early feeling

A colleague told me that during the first interview, when she felt invaded, she suspected psychosis in the patient. To illustrate this perceptual phenomenon, I will tell a story from my practice.

Many years ago, I received a man who told me about his difficulties, his obstacles in his professional life, and who wished to undertake a psychotherapy. After a few minutes of the interview, I felt an uncontrollable feeling of anxiety that persisted throughout the appointment and that challenged me: I waited to see him a second time to know if this anxiety was returning. It resurfaces in the same way. I take some time to think about it, I remember what the patient said, I reread my notes. I find nothing that can explain or justify my anxiety. His words are not threatening in any way, nothing that could make me anticipate a serious act and nothing in

6. Can psychiatric diagnosis be scientific?

his history that touches on painful points in me or in my past. The mystery of the anguish remains. I decide to talk about it to my controller, the one to whom the novice psychoanalyst talks about the difficulties encountered in his work. As I begin to describe the case I am confronted with, the diagnosis springs up: it is obviously a psychosis, even though this patient does not seem to resemble "a madman" in any way. The rest of the treatment will confirm the diagnosis. Unfortunately, my patient will sink into a schizophrenic state.

What conclusions can be drawn from this story? My anxiety reflected my early feeling about this patient, but this feeling was not conscious, it was replaced by affect. If it had been conscious I would probably have made a diagnosis of schizophrenia. An attempt was made to define this early feeling: it is the lack of empathy, the impossibility to get in touch with the patient, experienced in front of schizophrenics and autistics. This early feeling was related to listening, not to looking.

Schizophrenia, in its typical clinic, corresponds to a form, which makes some people say that "the secret of schizophrenia is a secret of the form[13]". I remember visiting a psychiatric hospital abroad and being struck by the fact that the schizophrenic patients at first glance resembled those I had treated in France. This non-individual form of schizophrenia suggests that clinical reasoning corresponds to the way, very well explained by neuroscience,

---

13. BOURGEOIS (Marc), RECHOULET (Danielle), "Les premières minutes, premier contact et rapidité diagnostique en psychiatrie", in Pierre Pichot and Werner Rein (under the direction of), *L'approche clinique en psychiatrie*, Paris, Les Empêcheurs de penser en rond, 1999.

in which a man recognizes another man, a table or any object. Apart from cases of cerebral pathologies leading to agnosia, the brain locates the characteristics of objects to recognize them, inferring them to a particular class. This process is perceptual in nature, commonplace and universal. Table types vary across cultures, but there is an invariant across cultural diversity. It is this invariant that is identified after being transmitted through language. In the same way, the clinic resembles a typology; but contrary to the spontaneous typology which allows us to recognize a bird or a cat, it is susceptible to confirmation as well as to reversal: it presents a critical aspect. The clinician identifies types, not stereotypes. It is then logical that the diagnosis can be rapid. When the picture deviates from the typical form, the clinician needs more time and has to rely on other less frequent data, because he does not see in what he observes an immediate family resemblance with the type in question. There are clinical cases that are completely prototypical and cases that deviate from the prototype. The German psychiatrist Kurt Schneider thought that the psychiatric symptom was not a sign as in somatic medicine, but a characteristic trait from which the observer could identify the type.

The limits of the integration of the medical method by the DSM

We can understand the intention of the designers of the DSM. They considered that this clinic, this way of making a diagnosis, lacked scientific rigor, that it was left to the vagaries of the clinician's subjectivity, that it hindered the progress of research and hindered the work of epidemiology and prevention because of its low reliability. They chose a method that allows for the most homogenization of patients' symptoms possible and that fits into a research protocol, but which requires sticking to accessible and easily observable behaviors.

The problem is that the DSM, which was based on criteria originally designed for research, has completely invaded the field of the clinic, which has distinct requirements. It must be admitted that there are several psychiatric clinics, which are heterogeneous to each other.

For example, if we learn that a patient considers himself to be worthless and useless, we can consider, if there are other signs, that he is suffering from depression and look for other symptoms that will validate the use of psychotropic drugs to treat him. But if we do not stick to the DSM method and we learn that it is not the first time that he feels this feeling of worthlessness, then we understand that it is a recurring feeling and we can look for connections between the situations and circumstances of life where this feeling of worthlessness was triggered. This does not prevent the patient from being prescribed a psychotropic drug, but it may be necessary to allow him to put his symptoms into perspective. Finally, if we learn that his mother also had similar thoughts, that he often heard her say that she felt worthless, we can consider that there is a family history, perhaps a genetic vulnerability, which reinforces the diagnosis of depression. We can also assume that this patient identifies with his depressed mother, which he refuses to admit, and that he rejects medication because he has seen his mother "take pills all her life," with no results.

I am trying to show at least two things with this example: on the one hand, the integration of clinical methods is tricky, because things somehow do not happen on the same scale, just as observation with the naked eye differs from observation with an ordinary microscope; on the other hand, if there was a time when the passion to classify had as a corollary the therapeutic impotence of classification and was only a game of the mind or a research without therapeutic repercussions, the classification of a case in such and such a pathology now carries consequences. Each pathological case is always a complex situation. Choices must be made, and this is precisely what the DSM method prevents. To use my metaphor of the microscope, it remains an observation with the naked eye, it is a surface observation without any depth of field, any perspective.

On the other hand, the clinical method, if it opens up a broader perspective allowing for in-depth work, also provides information. It allows for the collection of symptomatic data that can be useful in the context of rational drug prescription.

I am thinking in particular of a patient who was referred to me by her psychotherapist because she had perceived and heard that this patient was struggling with unusual affects. In fact, this patient was experiencing an overwhelming feeling of perplexity, synonymous with the onset of a delusional process that justified, in parallel with her psychotherapy, a prescription of neuroleptics. Another patient had had repeated depressive episodes from which he emerged without medication, but this time his analyst was alerted by a psychomotor slowdown that made him think that what was happening was not a simple repetition of previous episodes but something new that required a prescription of antidepressants.

These two examples show that the clinical approach, with its search for unconscious conflicts, does not systematically prevent a symptom-centered approach. Conversely, the DSM-based approach is so reductive that it makes anything other than medication or behavioral-cognitive therapy difficult or impossible.

This is one of the reasons for my hostility to the single DSM thought: by becoming the psychiatrist's mother tongue, it makes it very difficult for him to hear the polyphony of psychic life, the music of several rhythms and several tones of the symptoms. The clinical fact ends up escaping him. A psychiatrist must be able to change registers, and above all to play with the diversity of clinical approaches, but he still needs to have access to these different registers. The DSM plays the role of "ready-to-think", and forbids this diversity. The ideal, which does not exist, would be to have a clinical approach adapted to each case.

To conclude, I return to the original question: can diagnosis in psychiatry be scientific? My answer is no. The proof is in the DSM, which some people hailed as the entry of psychiatry into science or the modern era, with its criteria no longer based on "experience" but operational. Some people saw and greeted this paradigm shift with enthusiasm, but thirty years later, we must note the failures of this revolution, with the unprecedented impoverishment of the psychiatric corpus reduced to the description of everyday behaviors in order to pathologize them.

There is also what I have already mentioned several times because it is a serious problem for the health of the public: the DSM has allowed psychiatry to return to its inglorious past, that of triggering epidemics. There were several in the 19th century, including hysteria (with Charcot) and heredosyphilis, which turned out to be a chimera. Today, these epidemic triggers concern autism, attention deficit disorder with or without hyperactivity, and bipolar disorders, which appear to be a very reliable indicator of the absence of scientificity, despite the misplaced claims of certain DSM proponents. False epidemics are nosographic modes that take hold in the social field, first as a witness to a malaise in the culture, before becoming psychiatric categories to name this witness. If children seem to us to be more and more agitated, there are probably reasons for this, but it will be difficult to find them if we label them with a scientific pseudo-rationality. The name "index disorder" should be reserved for those who really are.

The DSM, however, has done more than revive the great epidemic eras. We are in an era where the stakes are about population control. Montesquieu understood that power tends to lead to abuse of power, that the enjoyment of power leads to "a little more power" and that his remedy was to limit power by other powers separated from each other: this is the brilliant principle of the separation of powers. What is true for the central power is also true for the "regional" powers, those of which Foucault speaks. Now, the psychiatric power, which is only a shadow of its former self, has kept the privilege of determining at least formally who is crazy and who is not, and this without the possible support of science. This is the diagnostic power. It uses and abuses this power by legislating who is ill and who is not, by extending its influence over the whole population, by facilitating the control of individuals. Hence the interest, as Montesquieu advocated, in bringing out other powers, other systems of classification, other approaches such as that of post-psychiatry, in advocating diversity in the absence of freedom of competition, which does not apply in this field.

Of course, the real power that would put an end to these excesses is the power of knowledge, of science, but there is nothing to indicate that the scientific era is near. Diagnosis in psychiatry is not scientific, the various clinical approaches are heterogeneous to each other, their integration in a single method is perhaps not possible, but this situation can lead to a positive synergy or to a passionate quarrel.

This will be the subject of my next chapter since I propose to talk about a controversial issue, that of autism; it illustrates perfectly how diagnostic and nosographic questions become important public health issues, with the participation of different actors, including of course the public authorities, but also a new force, a new power, that which is designated under the name of "mental health users".

7. The autism quarrel: disability versus madness

There have been many controversies and disputes, sometimes with a passionate tone, concerning the diagnosis and treatment of autistic people in recent years, and particularly in 2012. I will not repeat all the ideas that have been exchanged, but only focus on what is relevant to my topic, the DSM's fabrication of the insane.

A French deputy introduced a bill in which it was explained in substance that French child psychiatrists, referring to the French Classification of Mental Disorders of the Child and the Adolescent (CFTMEA), could not correctly diagnose autism, and especially could not treat it with adequate methods, this classification being of psychoanalytical orientation and assimilating autism to a mental pathology: "child psychosis". However, it has been proven that autism has an organic etiology, that it is a neurodevelopmental disorder, a distinction clearly established in foreign classifications such as the DSM or that of the World Health Organization (WHO), the ICD-10, which this deputy implied were more in line with science. He called for a ban on psychoanalytical practices with autistic people. Some time later, the French National Authority for Health (HAS) did not recommend psychoanalytical practices or institutional psychotherapy with autistic people, due to the lack of validated studies according to its criteria, which are based on what is called *Evidence Based Medicine (EBM)*. In other words, in the space of a few months, we have seen the emergence of an undertaking to invalidate both the French classification and psychoanalysis.

While this offensive removes the demeaning label of "crazy" from a population of children with disabilities, the problem is not just in these terms.

The changing perception of autism

After a long period of scientific history during which the wild child and then the idiots were described, autism was individualized by Leo Kanner in 1943 under the name of precocious infantile autism[14]. This syndrome presents two clinical features: extreme loneliness (*Aloneness*) and the need for immutability (*Sameless*). Kanner distin-

---

14. Kanner autism is the most severe form of autism.

guished autism from childhood schizophrenia, and his nosographic discovery was a turning point in child psychiatry because he focused on identifying the traits common to affected children, rather than looking for the signs described in adults. In this sense, his approach was innovative.

Then came a period when child psychiatrists and psychoanalysts, mostly English and French, set out to delimit the complex field of childhood psychoses in order to distinguish it from childhood schizophrenia, which was then "pervasive" in the United States. In particular, deficit psychoses (associated with mental retardation), dysthymic psychoses (associated with depressive episodes and possibly mania), symbiotic psychosis (manifested, among other things, by serious disturbances in social interactions), etc. were described. But early childhood autism retains its specificity. There are many reasons why psychoanalysts have linked autism to the field of psychoses, without including it. Among them, we must count the refusal of *the irreversibility* and *incurability* of autism by psychiatry at a certain time. Until psychoanalysis decided to invigorate the field of paedopsychiatry, which was encumbered by fixist theories.

Psychoanalysts have considered that autistic people have a defective psychic apparatus, and not only a defective brain, and they have tried to understand their functioning by comparing it with what they observed in psychoses. This resulted, for example, in clinical descriptions and hypotheses concerning the particular relationship of autistic people to objects, the question of the double, their relationship to language, the concepts of adhesive identification (mimetic identification) and projective identification (projection of the self onto the object), etc. All of these conceptual advances can be used in the service of an empathetic and therapeutic approach to autism, despite the great difficulties of care.

But the serious error of many psychoanalysts has been to promote explicitly or implicitly the idea that autism originates in the interaction between the child and the parents, and essentially in that with the mother. This "epistemological" option is erroneous and has in many cases been a source of suffering in addition to the suffering associated with autism itself.

In defence of the psychoanalysts, it should be said that the children were often referred to them at a late age and that they observed a clinical picture with a mother and a father at a distance, almost indifferent, and a child locked up in mutism. What they could not take into consideration were the very first moments of the child's life, when the parents had exhausted themselves stimulating the child, anxious, before becoming discouraged in front of the magnitude of the obstacle, all the more so as they did not find any help from the medical profession, insufficiently trained in this particular and specific question of infantile autism

Researchers have advanced the understanding of the autism clinic by proposing the installation of video cameras to film family moments in the first few months, such as baby's bath, meals, and all the main times of mother/baby exchange. Initially, the aim was to evaluate the quality and mechanisms of the mother/child bonding in order to understand possible deviations from the norm. The results showed that the vast majority of normal mothers faced with a child who did not respond normally went through successive phases that led to discouragement and psychological exhaustion. In these videos, it is striking to see, for example, a mother of identical twins, one of whom is normal and the other obviously autistic, behaving differently with the autistic child by over-stimulating him, anticipating responses that do not come, and mimicking a dialogue with him when in fact it is a monologue. With the normal twin, these attitudes and behaviors are not observed.

At the time of writing, the etiology of autism is not known. We know that there is a genetic involvement but we will not find the autism gene. We continue to search, in particular on the possible incidents during pregnancy. An increasingly insistent question, since the determination and delimitation of autism are still clinical: in the absence of biological markers, shouldn't "autism" be put in the plural? Are there not different types of autism that can be distinguished, for example, by the presence or absence of intellectual deficits? Is autism a well-defined syndrome or are there different syndromes? Is autism the final disabling pathway common to several different pathologies?

Autism as seen by the DSM

I obviously cannot answer all of these questions, but I will now focus on the implications of the DSM, how it addresses the problem and how it answers the nosographic questions of autism classification that I have just listed.

7. The autism quarrel: disability versus madness

Within the framework of thought reflected by the CFTMEA, we distinguish a gradient of pathology that goes from Kanner's autism, in its pure form, to the borderline states, passing through the autistic syndromes, the autistic reactions, and finally the infantile psychoses, called psychotic dysharmonies. It has even been described that certain exits from autism were made by passing through the infantile psychosis. However, this gradient has, in spite of itself, appeared to be a source of confusion and misunderstanding about a possible etiological, psychogenetic conception of autism. In the CFTMEA, child psychoses are used as a reference because of their reversible character and their accessibility to psychotherapeutic methods with a dynamic and mutative aim, without prejudging the other therapeutic, educational and pedagogical actions necessarily associated, and above all without taking sides for an etiology. However, the new rights offered by the status of disabled person, particularly in the United States, and the possibility of exculpation provided by the "universal" nature of science have converged to strongly influence the "modernization" of the nosographic conception of autism.

Autism, under the generic term of Pervasive Developmental Disorders (PDD), then Autism Spectrum Disorders (ASD) has become the absolute reference. Childhood psychoses have disappeared, and alongside a pure form of autism, we find other categories of PDD pathologies, which are defined negatively in relation to autism, as atypical or unspecified forms. The latter represent 35% of PDDs according to epidemiological studies, which suggests, on the one hand, that PDDs/ASDs are *chimerical groupings*, and, on the other hand, that these 35% correspond to the former childhood psychoses and borderline states or others, which, from constituted, characterized pathologies, and listed in the CFTMEA, are reduced to the confused status of "quasi-autism" or autism to this or that degree.

The confusion has changed sides, but the paradigms are no longer the same; it is the deficit conception and the handicap that are at the center. Asperger's syndrome continues to be a problem, as some dispute its deficit nature, without mentioning its blurred delimitations including "weird" people, schizoids or *borderlines.*

Another source of confusion is that mental retardation is rated only on Axis 2 of the DSM, which is the axis of incidental pathological features that do not qualify for pathological status. But since the parents of these mentally retarded children are demanding a *true diagnosis* on axis 1 - that of true pathologies - mental retardation is included in PDD/ASD. The DSM-5 finally retained Asperger's Syndrome as part of ASD and removed the axes, thus solving the problem of the status of mental disabilities. The pendulum has shifted in favour of disability, a change that has been endorsed by legislators for several years.

How the DSM freezes all childhood psychoses as disabilities

Fighting to have a syndrome previously considered a mental pathology recognized as a disability is perfectly

7. The autism quarrel: disability versus madness

understandable, especially since the word psychosis is stigmatizing. Telling parents "your child is psychotic" is equivalent to telling them "your child is crazy", which is terrible for a child and makes parents feel guilty; it is easy to imagine that they will ask themselves the question of their responsibility in the emergence of their child's madness and as there is no scientific explanation, they will remain with this insistent question. If they are told "your child is handicapped", the statement will provoke other reactions but the conscious guilt will be less solicited. However, will they have gained anything at all?

In my experience of working with mentally handicapped children and their parents, regardless of the diagnosis or the words used, it is important to know how to collect their guilt. Parents experience this guilt as soon as the disability is announced, and even before, when the disorders are identified. What are the usual contents of this feeling of guilt? "I could not protect my child", "I passed on a defect in spite of myself", etc. The simple fact of bringing a child "like no other" into the world generates a feeling of guilt. It is important to respect this guilt, without ever aggravating it and without fighting it directly, because it is also the mark of parental involvement, it is co-extensive or inherent to all parenthood.

I reject the idea of an a priori standardized response to the guilt of parents of mentally handicapped children, but it may be useful to state, for example, that any child, regardless of the degree or extent of his or her handicap, is likely to learn, and that it is beneficial to note with some emphasis the emergence of a new skill in the child. It is recognized, even by some critics of psychoanalysis, that psychoanalysts are often best trained to take on the task of talking with parents. Faced with the weight of this "irremediable", the psychiatrist can nevertheless play a positive role by explaining that there is always potential for the child to evolve, even if it is very small. There are strategies and techniques to compensate for the handicap, and the psychiatrist can help to link mutation and compensation.

The disabled child, like the normal child, is inscribed in the fantasy of the parents, who want the child to be like this or like that, to correspond to this or that norm or ideal. They want to be proud of it, that it compensates for certain lacks, certain failures, etc. But the disabled child hurts the parents' self-image and self-esteem. I would say that it produces a narcissistic wound, especially if it presents visible deformities that can evoke monstrosity. But the reaction is not always the same; I remember a meeting of parents of handicapped children where the mother of a Down's syndrome boy asked why the teachers of the center where her son was admitted did not take class photos so that the children could keep a souvenir; she pointed out that her son had felt in trouble when, one afternoon, his brothers and sisters had shown each other their class photos. Then another mother of a child with Down syndrome spoke up and said that the class photo was a bad idea: she didn't want to expose or have exposed in a photo her son's disability, she already suffered enough from the looks of others when she was on the street or on the bus with him. He would lower his head when someone stared at him and she was ashamed. The first mother replied, "But you have to teach them to

7. The autism quarrel: disability versus madness

defend themselves, ma'am. I, my son, the other day, a tall teenager was staring at him on the bus... Well, he held that teenager's gaze and he said to her in a threatening way, "Do you want my picture?""

This mother had managed to overcome her narcissistic wound. This story is likely, it seems to me, to make us understand how each case is particular, how reactions differ from one family to another, but also the interest of discussion groups between parents of disabled children. I am convinced that this reflection on the fact that children must be taught to defend themselves had more impact on the other mother than if it had been said by the educators, the psychologist or any other professional, because it came from a parent living a comparable experience. Parents of mentally handicapped children have much to teach us about the fragility of the social bond and about the norm.

I now return, after this detour, to a question that is increasingly present in the field of autism and in child psychiatry in general: what is the relationship between mental illness and disability and what role does the DSM play in this debate? I think that the DSM and the ICD, by their deficit conception and their implicit organicist presuppositions, have led to an artificial separation between handicap and pathology, a separation that was ratified by the 2005 law on autism, which defines autism as a handicap. Their conception resembles a return to the old fixist theories but is now associated with behavioralist compensation techniques promoted by studies with contested results (by scientists who are not suspected of complacency towards psychoanalysis) and by an aggressive strategy resembling marketing. The therapeutic results of these techniques are real, but here again it is necessary to qualify them, because in a number of studies there are children labelled as "unspecified autism"; however, taking into account what I have already said, it would appear that they are in reality, camouflaged under this "label", former infantile psychoses, which we know are very often reversible.

The designers of the CFTMEA, and Roger Misès in the first place, refused this separation pathology/disability, because, they said, mental pathologies lead to handicaps that are sometimes severe, and, conversely, the persistence of disadvantages in social interactions contribute to the fixation of psychopathological mechanisms that are sometimes very constraining. Hence, whenever possible, the need for caregivers to encourage a convergence and a positive synergy instead of a separation between structural changes and progress made in the field of school, family or later social adaptation. The CFTMEA is accompanied by a classification of disabilities within the framework of Philip Wood's dynamic conceptions[15]. This dynamic conception between disability and pathology is confirmed by the work on brain-injured people, which demonstrates the accuracy of a functional approach to disability: any cerebral deficit following an injury leads to a strategy of compensation of this deficit by the organism. The result is that the symptoms are not only related

---

15. Philip Wood (1928-2008) was a British epidemiologist and rheumatologist who changed the view of disability by defining it as a disadvantage in fulfilling a social role due to impairment or disability.

to the deficit but also to the deficit and the compensation mechanisms implemented by the brain.

Research avenues are opening up for autism. For example, when psychoanalysts speak of an autistic-type defense mechanism, is it an unconscious defense mechanism, with or without intentionality, against "an unbearable reality?" Of an unconscious fantasy? Of impulses? Or a strategy of compensation of the failing brain of the autistic person?

The question of autism is a difficult one and is at the crossroads of many epistemological and theoretical issues, but also of public health and finance. I am in favor of an integrative and multidisciplinary approach to autism that puts aside ideological quarrels, because the psychoanalytical approach no longer exists and the rehabilitative approach is ethically questionable. I will make my point more precisely: the DSM produces, in the same movement, more and more "false mad" children to be calmed and controlled, and, in the name of an ideal mixing political correctness and scientism, it only sees handicapped people who all belong to ASD. This last choice was not only made against psychoanalysis, but also by neglecting valuable works such as those of the Yale School, which rightly speaks of *multiple complex development disorder*. In both cases, there is a distortion of reality and it goes against common sense, but it testifies once again to the extent to which the diagnostic categories, the different headings of the psychiatric classifications are nothing but historically dated social constructions.

8. Resistance to the DSM: a social issue

As early as the 1980s, while many psychiatrists welcomed the revolution that the release of the DSM-3 represented in their eyes, others welcomed it with indifference, and others began to resist. Among the DSM-3 supporters, there was no homogeneity. Some psychiatrists had suffered from feeling devalued by the psychoanalytic approach, either because they were not psychoanalysts themselves, or because they did not accept what appeared to them to be a single way of thinking, or finally because they were scientifically minded and the scientific nature of psychoanalysis seemed dubious.

The desire to make psychoanalysis a science at all costs

This opinion could have been reinforced by the work of Adolf Grünbaum who had tried in several works to demonstrate, with a solid and structured argument, that basic Freudian concepts, such as repression, could not reach the status of scientific concept. Adolf Grünbaum follows Karl Popper, even if he disagrees with him. Popper reproached psychoanalysis for producing unfalsifiable statements; however, the mark of scientific theories is that they lend themselves to refutation. In other words, psychoanalysis cannot claim to be scientific. Karl Popper's other argument is the fact that psychoanalysis has the vocation or claim to explain everything. But, he says, when a theory explains everything, it explains nothing. He writes, in *L'Univers irrésolu : plaidoyer pour l'indéterminisme* : "Insofar as the propositions of science relate to reality, they are not certain, and insofar as they are certain they do not relate to reality". This propensity of psychoanalysis to explain everything has been seen at work in the field of psychoses and in the field of autism. It is understandable that it has profoundly annoyed certain logical or scientific minds, especially if they were confronted with the argument of "their resistance to psychoanalysis". But in reality, there are serious answers to the objection that psychoanalysis is not scientific, Freud himself had tackled this in a famous article, *Constructions in Analysis*[16]. But to list all the arguments

---

16. FREUD (Sigmund), "Constructions in Analysis", *Results, Ideas, Problems*, vol. 2, 1921-1938, Paris, Presses universitaires de France, 1998.

would be to take me away from my subject. In any case, in our time, demonstrating that a theory is not scientific is a ruinous argument for this theory, which is relegated to the rank of false theory or religion. One question remains, however: how is it that the argument of non-scientific nature has been able to carry the day when it comes to psychoanalysis, whereas it does not seem to harm in the same proportions when it is addressed to the DSM methodology, which is no more scientific?

My explanation lies in the fact that psychoanalysis is perceived as the bearer of truths, even if they are applied on a case-by-case basis and require the passage through the cure, whereas the DSM methodology claims to be atheoretical - so as not to expose itself head-on to epis-temological criticism - while having the contours of what Canguilhem calls a scientific ideology, i.e. a belief that squints at a science by imitating it without being scien-tific. In this case it is a mixture of sciences. Moreover, the methodology of the DSM based on operational criteria has a family resemblance with truth, it follows the scien-tific zeitgeist and it is known that sometimes theories that only had an air of truth have been proven true later on. Hence the weak impact of the DSM critique on the terrain of scientificity.

The professional body of psychiatrists, as I have already said, has found itself locked in with its patients. Some of them do not complain about it, they accept this confinement in the name of specificity. They are in a deliberate ghetto posture. Others have never accepted it; this posture seems to them to have been imposed. For the latter, the DSM-3 was a real godsend, a liberating document that allowed them to speak as equals with their somatic colleagues. But if there is no longer a psychological reality, only a cerebral reality, psychopathology disappears and with it psychiatry as distinct from neurology.

This was the hope of some, but it turned out to be an imaginary neurology. The biological markers that were "coming soon" were overdue. From announcements to bluffing or "commercial swindles", hope was maintained. This Messiah was for tomorrow, he would free psychiatry from its magical prescientific ornaments and at the same time make the psychiatrist an authentic doctor, an authentic man of science.

The expectation of belief has passed a little among psychiatrists, but it is still very much present in the press, which disseminates research work in its own way, and above all in the public, among the users of psychiatry, first and foremost patients and their families. In reality, no decisive step in the understanding of the cause of mental illnesses has been taken in the last thirty years, although it is regularly announced in magazines and especially in newspaper articles that we are on the way to discovering the gene for autism, the gene for alcoholism, the gene for schizophrenia or the gene for depression. It is true that, for some time now, after the catchy title, in the body of the article, one can read much more nuanced statements and, in general, as the popular expression goes, the mountain gives birth to a mouse.

The fight against the DSM, the bible of American psychiatry

From the outset, a certain number of thinkers, especially European thinkers[17], were concerned about the DSM. They saw it as a symptom of our cultural malaise, but their point of view was mainly moral, or rather political in the broad sense of the term, denouncing the ethical deficit to which the DSM testifies, and the anthropological change that it would accompany. Their criticism, however relevant, has unfortunately not had a significant impact, because on the other side of the Atlantic, people are not as sensitive to ethical questioning. People are generally reluctant to be satisfied with an aerial view, however brilliant it may be. Then, little by little, a number of Americans began to undermine the authority of the DSM. They pointed out the "side effects" of the DSM in the daily reality of Americans. I am thinking of Stuart Kirk and Herb Kutchins' book, *Do* you *like the DSM?*[18]. They begin with the disaster that the use of the DSM is causing in the field of psychiatric expertise. It is a resistance that is conceptual, intellectual, but based on concrete examples. Its impact has been greater because it speaks to people who may be concerned in many ways: personal mental illness or affecting loved ones, psychiatric exper-

---

17. I am thinking in particular of the historian and psychoanalyst Elisabeth Roudinesco, the psychoanalyst Roland Gori and the psychiatrist and psychoanalyst Maurice Corcos.

18. Kirk (Stuart), Kutchins (Herb), *Aimez-vous le DSM ? Le triomphe de la psychiatrie américaine*, Paris, Les Empêcheurs de tourner en rond, 1998.

8. Resistance to the DSM: a social issue

tise in the case of criminal or even civil litigation, in the case of divorce for the custody of children or even in the case of guardianship or curatorship.

In fact, what is striking about reading the critiques of the DSM in the United States is the scope of the DSM, its reach beyond drug prescriptions, which has led to the claim that the DSM is the bible of American psychiatry. This "sacred" status may be the reason why the DSM has become so popular with Hollywood screenwriters. DSM language appears in a lot of movie dialogue, especially between young characters. The DSM-3 was a totally unexpected bestseller that filled the coffers of the American Psychiatric Association and proved that it met an expectation.

Mental illness, but also mental functioning in general, is of interest to everyone and the DSM offers the general public the opportunity to learn about psychiatry. The DSM is psychiatry for dummies. It is becoming a social phenomenon, the language of psychiatry is becoming part of everyday life as well as the possibility of self-expertise. Certain "psychoanalytical" expressions have also invaded everyday language. I am thinking of the expression "mourning", the content of which is relatively vague, but about which a lawyer friend of mine told me that this expression is sometimes used in the courts, in particular when a civil party's lawyer claims that the sentence requested by the prosecution is not sufficient for the victim to begin her mourning process, or that the compensation is too low, etc. But this contamination is limited, it only concerns certain very specific expressions; whereas there is a wide diffusion of the DSM language among the general public: "I suffer from OCD", "I am bipolar", etc.

American psychoanalysts have resisted the DSM-3 in several ways. Some of them sulked about it and refused to take part in the project, others played along but had to jump ship because they felt that it was a trap, that the orientation of the decision-makers was fundamentally opposed to psychoanalysis. Around the year 2000, American psychoanalysts, together with a few international personalities such as Daniel Widlöcher, sought a new response to the DSM. They designed a manual entitled *Psychodynamic Diagnostic Manual (PDM)* which was intended to be a complement to the DSM, a sixth axis[19] psychopathology. They conducted studies proving the effectiveness of psychoanalysis and analytical psychotherapies. They applied evaluation criteria from *Evidence Based Medicine* to psychodynamic psychotherapy, transforming these psychotherapies into *Empirically Supported Therapy*. By this concession to American positivism, they have opened the way to a field of research on the evaluation of psychotherapies, a delicate path because evaluation and psychoanalysis do not mix well.

There are also the criticisms of the DSM which focus on its impact on mental health, on false epidemics, on

---

19. The DSM is composed of five axes: Axis 1 focuses on major clinical disorders; Axis 2 on personality disorders and mental retardation; Axis 3 on specific medical aspects and physical disorders; Axis 4 on psycho-social and environmental factors; and finally, Axis 5, called the "Global Assessment of Functioning" scale, assesses the individual's psychological, social and occupational functioning.

8. Resistance to the DSM: a social issue

the medicalization of emotions and existence, on over-diagnosis, over-prescription, and the manufacture of madmen[20], which I share.

The question of the DSM is also that of American positivism, that is to say, a way of thinking, a philosophy that advocates that knowledge is only acquired through experience. However, it was necessary to wait until people had experienced the DSM before they were receptive to its critique and even to its radical critique; they could not be satisfied with an a priori critique on ethical or political grounds. Positivism has values, such as reality, efficiency, usefulness, experimentation, certainty, and for a critique of the DSM to be effective, not to remain confidential, it must integrate these values. This is what is currently happening among the associations or critical movements in the United States. Never before has an edition of the DSM aroused so much opposition and so many numerical arguments as version 5. It is not impossible that this will be the last edition and that we will be able to say goodbye to the DSM, because the system has almost imploded under the effect of internal and external criticism. This disappearance will not be regrettable, but what will replace the DSM?

It is this question that led me to engage with a dozen or so fellow analysts belonging to all the psychoanalytic associations in an action against the single thought DSM. This action led us to write a manifesto that gathered thousands of signatures, to organize two Stop DSM days in Paris. We created the association Initiative pour une

---

20. See in particular the work of Christopher Lane and Allen Frances.

Clinique du Sujet. Our action, which has received a favorable echo in the Hispanic and Anglo-Saxon world, is based on three axes: a well-founded refusal of the DSM methodology, political action with decision-makers to alert them to the dangers of the DSM, and action with the media to inform and raise public awareness. Finally, Roger Misès, this pioneer of the anti-DSM struggle, took the initiative, before leaving us, to set up with the psychiatrist Jean Garrabé a working group to elaborate a classification of adult mental illnesses on the same model as the CFTMEA, which I have already mentioned.

All these initiatives, all these collective or individual actions coming from different horizons are meant to show that there is a resistance to the DSM that is not satisfied with denouncing and petitioning, but that proposes other methods. It is not a question of locking ourselves into a posture of indignation against the DSM, but perhaps of opening the way to a new period, which breaks with reductionism and fixism, and which can offer an alternative classification useful for the transmission of clinical knowledge to young practitioners. After the Stop DSM period, we must prepare for the post-DSM period, which will put an end to the diagnostic inflation that makes people see crazy people everywhere.

Conclusion

At the end of this work, there remains an objection to which I have not responded: that of conservatism.

I can indeed be reproached for refusing modernization and simplification, for refusing to change, which I would defend with great arguments; for draping myself in my ethical dignity; for being a dinosaur fit for Jurassic Park. One might add that this resistance to the DSM by a certain number of psychoanalysts is nothing more than a resistance to biological psychiatry and neuroscience; a reaction of a has-been who does not want to recognize that his knowledge has gone out of fashion and that a new, more efficient technology has now entered his field.

There is undoubtedly some truth in this criticism, especially if we refer to the decade 1990-2000. At that time, the DSM had the look of new technology, it had introduced or helped to introduce into the field of subjectivity instruments, tools that were more objective, simpler, less intuitive, more assessable, and more easily transmissible. Moreover, it had helped to reduce the gap between clinical and research, a gap that is a cause of obstacles to progress in the discipline. Moreover, the DSM, by basing itself on *Evidence Based Medicine*, opened the way and above all favoured the era of evaluation in psychiatry, which was the last place in medicine where managerial efficiency was difficult to enter. For some it is a disaster, for others a blessing.

Even if we do not reject the idea of evaluating care, we cannot accept that the teaching and practice of psychiatry be done with the same instrument as that used for managerial efficiency. The role of health manager is not the role of psychiatrist. There must be a transcoding between the two practices: the clinician reasons with his clinical concepts, he produces a diagnosis in the logic of his code, which must be translated into another code, for administrative use. Otherwise, it is the language of Babel, with a single, even totalitarian aim.

So to the objection that might be directed at me, I would say: The DSM is a success story of coding, but is coding always progress? Is the DSM code only a modernization of the old clinic and a scientific simplification? Codification is in itself a rationalization undertaking, but not every rationalization undertaking is necessarily useful or necessarily scientific. The DSM code is based on operational criteria for pharmacological research, the usefulness of which I do not dispute, of course, but this is only one area of psychiatry. Psychopharmacological research does not aim to represent or encompass all psychiatric practices, but this choice is far from neutral; by taking the criteria useful for research as a reference, the patient of the clinic is replaced by the target patient of psychotropic drugs. The reference model is the "chemical" patient, the "neuronal man[21]". By taking this patient as the standard, the DSM has shifted the center of gravity of previous psychiatric classifications and manuals. It is therefore not a simple codification but a change of reference. This change could have been justified if the neural model had allowed decisive advances in the study of the mechanisms involved in mental pathologies. However, at the time when the DSM-3 was conceived, these advances did not exist; they were hoped for. This is what I have ironically called the "believing expectation". The change was therefore a gamble on the future. We know that this bet has since been lost. The DSM was based on a fiction, or rather a science fiction.

The neurochemical patient was a Trojan horse for the pharmaceutical industry, which took advantage of the unexpected opportunity offered by the American Psychiatric Association. It allowed itself to manufacture, or rather to "help manufacture", diagnoses that could be targets for the drugs it produced. In this respect, the circumstances of the "invention" of social phobia[22] is

---

21. Formula of Jacques-Alain Miller, taken up by Changeux (Jean-Pierre), *L'Homme neuronal*, Paris, Fayard, coll. "Le temps des sciences", 1983.
22. See LANE (Christopher), *Comment la psychiatrie et l'industrie phar-maceutique ont médicalisé nos émotions*, Paris, Flammarion, coll. "La Bibliothèque des Savoirs", 2009.

paradigmatic of the "new method" which consists of an inversion of the usual method: whereas one was looking for the adequate treatment for a proven disease, one now manufactures the target syndrome to which a treatment already found will correspond.

There is another important aspect to this Herculean codification undertaking that the DSM-3 and its subsequent editions represented. A code serves to enact rules: take the famous Code Napoléon, or Civil Code, whose stability and longevity have been remarkable, what goal did the jurists of the time have assigned to themselves by the Emperor? To enact identical rules throughout France, to unify the various customs into a single code in order to achieve national unity and equality of citizens before the law. The Civil Code governs civil life, which is everyday life. So what about the DSM code? As I said, it takes as reference the neurochemical man. As psychotropic drugs act on our emotions and behaviours, the idea of codifying emotions and behaviours naturally imposed itself on the promoters of the DSM. Initially, it was only a matter of identifying and observing pathological behaviours and emotions, but it came to codify these emotions and behaviours, i.e., to legislate what is a normal behaviour and what is not, what is a normal emotion and what is not. Who is the "legislator" of this code of emotions and behaviors? It is the consensus of the psychiatrists and experts who work on the DSM. This can be seen as an incredible re-establishment of psychiatric power, because giving a professional group the power to legislate on our behaviours and emotions is tantamount to the State delegating regulatory power to it, and to civil society submitting to this power: any citizen in the United States can have the norms laid down by the DSM set against him or her by a judge.

We are all concerned by the DSM, and it is necessary to think twice before introducing it as the only reference in France, a serious risk because of its transcultural vocation and the influence of the United States. It has the universal status of science and its prestige, despite its deceptions.

The word "normal" entered the French political scene in 2012, during the televised debate between the remaining candidates in the second round of the presidential campaign. This entry bodes well, as everyone understood that whoever used it was doing so with the idea that everyone knew what normal was. There is a sense of justice very early in a child's life, educators tell us. There may also be an intuitive sense of normal in everyone, but the difficulty is that neurochemical man has a variable geometry normality that is not measured on biological constants but on behaviors and emotions. Unless the norm is "zero emotions and perfect behavior".

The real question, dear reader, is whether you are willing to submit to a code of civility or civilization, because the moral dimension is never far away when codifying the behaviors enacted by the American Psychiatric Association or any other psychiatric association.

It was my ambition in writing this book to try to enlighten your opinion.

Acknowledgements

To Jack Carney, Allen Frances, Jean Garrabé, Peter Kinderman, Christopher Lane.

To the members of the association Initiative pour une Clinique du Sujet :

Jean-Caude Aguerre, Guy Dana, Marielle David, Francis Drossard, Françoise Fabre, Tristan Garcia-Fons, Nicolas Gougoulis, Thierry Jean, Claude Léger, François Leguil, Geneviève Nusinovici, Bernard Odier, Michel Patris, Gérard Pommier, Jean-François Solal, Dominique Tourrès, Jean-Jacques Tyszler, Alain Vanier

To those who participate in CFTMA:
Marcianne Blévis, Michel Botbol, Aurélie Capobianco, Laurent Delhommeau, Olivier Douville, Bernard Gibello, François Kammerer, Jean-Baptiste Legouis, Nora Markman, Claire Nahon, Frédéric Pellion, Christian Portelli, Dominique Wintrebert

Table of contents

Best sellers Max Milo Editions

Hitler's banker, Jean-François Bouchard

Confessions of a forger, Éric Piedoie Le Tiec

The Koran and the flesh, Ludovic-Mohamed Zahed

Governing by fake news, Jacques Baud

Governing by chaos, Collectif

A political history of food, Paul Ariès

Mad in U.S.A.: The ravages of the "American model",
Michel Desmurget

Mondial soccer club geopolitics, Kévin Veyssière

Putin: Game master?, Jacques Braud

Treatise on the three impostors: Moses, Jesus, Muhammad,
The Spirit of Spinoza

TV Lobotomy, Michel Desmurget